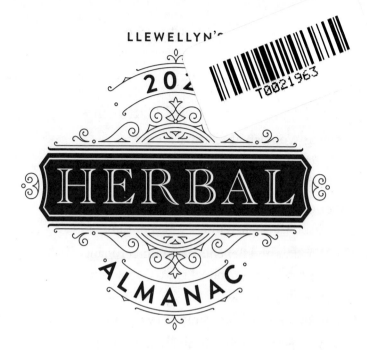

LLEWELLYN'S

2025

HERBAL

ALMANAC

Llewellyn's 2025 Herbal Almanac Copyright © 2024 Llewellyn
Worldwide Ltd. All rights reserved.
ISBN: 978-0-7387-7193-9

Cover Design by Kevin R. Brown
Editing and layout by Lauryn Heineman
Interior illustrations by Llewellyn Art Department

You can order annuals and books from *New Worlds,*
Llewellyn's catalog. To request a free copy, call 1-877-
NEW WRLD toll-free or visit www.llewellyn.com.

Llewellyn Worldwide Ltd.
2143 Wooddale Drive
Woodbury, MN 55125-2989

Printed in China

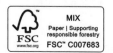

MIX
Paper | Supporting
responsible forestry
FSC™ C007683
FSC
www.fsc.org

Contents

Health and Beauty

DIY and Crafts

Plant Profiles

Gardening Resources

Introduction to
Llewellyn's Herbal Almanac

Holistic care for the mind, body, and soul starts in the garden. While adapting to the new normal, people around the world have sought out sustainable lifestyles and made greener choices, asking how to grow and preserve organic food for their family or how to forage for a nutritious bounty in their own neighborhood. Growing herbs enriches the soul, and using them in home-cooked meals, remedies, and crafts is natural, healthy, and just plain delicious.

There is no better time to grow, use, and eat herbs than now, and we hope you'll find inspiration for your own healthy life in this book. With sage advice appealing to novice gardeners and experienced herbalists alike, our experts tap into the practical and historical aspects of herbal knowledge—using herbs to help you connect with the earth, enhance your culinary creations, and heal your body and mind.

In addition to the twenty-four articles written by Master Gardeners, nutritionists, homesteaders, and community herbalists, this book offers reference materials tailored specifically for successful growing and gathering. Use this book to plot this year's garden, practice companion planting, learn a new cooking technique, garden by the moon, find a helpful herbal remedy, and keep track of goals and chores.

Reclaiming our connection to Mother Earth in our own backyards can bring us harmony and balance—and a delicious, healthy harvest. May your garden grow lush and your dishes taste divine!

Note: The old-fashioned remedies in this book are historical references used for teaching purposes only. The recipes are not for commercial use or profit. The contents are not meant to diagnose, treat, prescribe, or substitute consultation with a licensed healthcare professional. Herbs, whether used internally or externally, should be introduced in small amounts to allow the body to adjust and to detect possible allergies. Please consult a standard reference source or an expert herbalist to learn more about the possible effects of certain herbs. You must take care not to replace regular medical treatment with the use of herbs. Herbal treatment is intended primarily to complement modern healthcare. Always seek professional help if you suffer from illness. Also, take care to read all warning labels before taking any herbs or starting on an extended herbal regimen. Always consult medical and herbal professionals before beginning any sort of medical treatment—this is particularly true for pregnant women. Herbs are powerful things; be sure you are using that power to achieve balance.

Llewellyn Worldwide does not participate in, endorse, or have any authority or responsibility concerning private business transactions between its authors and the public.

Growing
and
Gathering

Growing Woodland Medicinal Herbs

⊱ Jordan Charbonneau ⊰

For many herbalists, the herbs we reach for are the ones we first learned to identify in our yards and gardens. Some are familiar childhood weeds like dandelion, while others like echinacea and chamomile find their places in our gardens as we develop our craft. However, there are several potent medicinal herbs that don't grow in our sunny gardens; instead, they're hidden away in cool hollers, forested mountainsides, and winding ridges. Many of these woodland herbs were first gathered and used by Indigenous peoples who passed some of their knowledge on to colonists settling these areas.

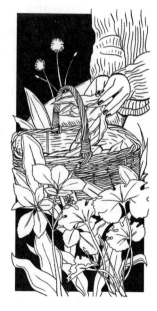

Native peoples, settlers, and their descendants relied on these woodland herbs to remedy various ailments and illnesses, often where doctors were too expensive or difficult to reach. Some of these herbs also began supporting mountain folk in other ways.

Perhaps no woodland medicinal herb has as rich a commercial history as American ginseng (*Panax quinquefolius*), which has been wild-harvested for commercial sale for over 250 years. In the 1700s, it "made history as one of the first US products exported to China," reports Alex Schechter for Vox. Today, ginseng and several other American woodland herbs remain highly sought-after. Probably the most lucrative, ginseng can go for between $500 and $1,000 per pound, notes Emily Cataneo for *Wired*.

While less valuable than ginseng, bloodroot, goldenseal ("yellow root" to some Appalachian families), ramps, and a few others share a long history of commercial harvesting and use.

Though the prices of these herbs may sound like a great boon to rural herbal folk, the reality is far from it. Generally, the companies purchasing these herbs only want wild-harvested herbs, taxing already strained populations. They also pay the diggers, often people from economically depressed, rural communities, pennies on the dollar.

Thankfully, if you have just a small patch of woods, you can easily take a step back from these exploitive companies and help preserve some incredible species by planting your own.

Native Woodland Medicinal Herbs and Their Benefits

There are numerous woodland herbs that you can propagate. Many of those that are the most highly sought-after are also the most at risk. The United Plant Savers offers an up-to-date list of endangered and at-risk herbs. Here are a few considered at risk, which you may want to cultivate on your property.

American Ginseng (*Panax quinquefolius*)

Few plants carry ginseng's history and lore. Widely known in the herbal world as a powerful adaptogen, Asian ginseng has a history of use dating back thousands of years. The Chinese *The Divine Husbandman's Classic of the Materia Medica*, dating to the first century CE, mentions using ginseng medically. In North America, American ginseng's use also has a long history. Native peoples, including the Cherokee, used the herb as a stimulant and to treat headaches, colds, infertility, and congestion.

Today, this inconspicuous herbaceous perennial plant remains an important, valued herb. American ginseng is protected under state and federal laws. In many areas, a permit is required to harvest this plant or its seed anywhere but your own land. There is also a regulated season for ginseng. Poaching ginseng is illegal in many areas and is a felony in North Carolina.

American ginseng comes up in spring, usually in April. One-year-old plants feature three leaflets that join together on a two-to-four-inch stalk. During this first year, the plant begins forming a small fleshy root with a bud near the top. In the fall, ginseng goes dormant, and the leaves and stem turn yellow and then die back for the winter.

A new stem emerges from the bud in spring. Each year the plant grows bigger and grows more prongs of compound leaves. Two-year-old plants generally have two compound leaves, each with five to seven ovate leaflets. At this stage, the stem is typically four to seven inches tall. In subsequent years the plant may develop three to (rarely) five prongs of compound leaves and reach heights of twelve to twenty-four inches.

After a ginseng plant is three years old or more, it will begin producing seed. In midsummer, it develops greenish flowers, which form small green berries that ripen to red in late summer. Each berry contains two to four seeds.

In many areas, wild ginseng plants must have three prongs to harvest legally. Ideally, this ensures the plant has produced some seed and offspring before being harvested. While you may legally harvest your own ginseng at any time, it's best to wait until it is mature and has seeded new plants.

Goldenseal (*Hydrastis canadensis*)

Goldenseal is another beloved and commercially valued herb. In my neck of the woods, many refer to this plant as yellow root, although it should be noted that other plants share that common name. It's valued for its two major alkaloids, hydrastine and berberine. It's the berberine that gives the roots their bright yellow coloring and bitter flavor.

Native Americans, including the Cherokee and Iroquois, used goldenseal as medicine and dye long before colonists came to North America. Modern herbalists sometimes employ goldenseal to treat sore throats, coughs, mouth sores, nasal congestion, giardiasis, and hemorrhoids.

Goldenseal is a perennial herbaceous herb. In the spring, the plant produces a flowering stem with two large hairy leaves. The leaves are palmate and may be up to twelve inches wide and eight inches long with prominent veins and five to seven lobes. The plant features small, inconspicuous flowers in late spring, which lack petals and instead have many white

About half of the woodland plants and plant parts sold as part of the billion-dollar herbal products industry are native to Appalachia and are part of a long history of industries taking Appalachia's resources without returning money to local communities, according to faculty and students of Virginia Tech.

stamens surrounding the pistil. The flower gives way to a single fruit that ripens to red and appears like a red raspberry at first glance. The fruit contains ten to twenty-five seeds.

Like ginseng, goldenseal's most valued part is its root, which is actually a horizontal rhizome. The rhizome may be one-half to three-quarter inch thick and is covered in fibrous roots. The roots and rhizome are bright yellow; it's easily noticeable if you break one.

Bloodroot (*Sanguinaria canadensis*)

The pattern of a long history of traditional use followed by commercial overharvesting, as discussed for the previous two herbs, continues with bloodroot. Native peoples used this plant for thousands of years as a natural dye and in medicinal preparations for various ailments, including respiratory, gastrointestinal, and skin issues. European colonists were quick to add bloodroot into their own medicinal practices. The plant was officially listed in the United States Pharmacopeia in 1820. However, it can have some very negative side effects, even when used externally. For that reason, modern herbalists consider it to be an expert-only herb. If you're unfamiliar, consult a knowledgeable herbalist.

Bloodroot is what's known as a **spring ephemeral**. The stem and leaves die back in the fall, and in very early spring, a single white flower with a yellow center appears. The flower grows on a single stem two to four inches tall that's wrapped in folded leaves. The leaves unfurl as the flower blooms. The leaves are green above and pale below, with many lobes and undulating margins. Their undersides are noticeably veined, and as they unfurl to their full size, they may reach about nine inches wide.

After the flower is pollinated and fades, the flower stem elongates and forms a green seed pod containing ten to fifteen seeds. When the seeds are ripe, the pod splits open and releases the seeds, each with a fleshy organ called an **elaiosome**. This organ attracts native ants, which take the seeds, eat the elaiosome, and then bury the unharmed seed in their trash dump, where it will eventually grow. Unfortunately, non-native ants damage both the elaiosome and the seed. The spread of non-native ants has contributed to the plant's decline.

Bloodroot is named and known for its horizontal underground rhizome, which features bright red or dark orange sap when broken. The rhizome grows about one-half inch thick and up to four inches long. It eventually branches to form a colony.

Ramps (*Allium tricoccum*)

Ramps are the smelliest and tastiest herb on this list with their pungent onion- or garlic-like flavor and odor. They are a beloved wild food throughout their range, and you may have spotted these flavor-packed spring delicacies at your local farmers' market. In Appalachia, they're so popular that there are even festivals dedicated to them! Unfortunately, this has led to widespread overharvesting and has earned them a spot on the at-risk plant list.

Beyond their flavor, ramps have been historically valued for their medicinal and nutritional properties. Ramps are one of the first wild edibles collected en masse in early spring and were an essential source of vitamins for those living on the edge of survival in the mountains. Native Americans including the Ojibwa, Cherokee, and Iroquois incorporated ramps into their medicinal practices, using them as a spring tonic and to treat conditions like colds, flu, worms, and respiratory ailments.

Ramps are spring ephemerals, dying back in the winter and sending up two to three green elliptic or lanceolate leaves that look a bit like young tulip leaves in the spring. When torn or crushed, their intense oniony odor easily distinguishes them as a member of the allium family. The leaves may be purple-tinged near the base, may have a papery sheath, and can reach eight inches tall. Like other onion family members, the leaves grow from a small whitish bulb. Both the bulbs and the leaves are edible.

The leaves die back as surrounding trees leaf out, and then in early summer, the plant sends up a flower stalk with umbels of creamy white to greenish flowers. After pollination, each flower gives way to a small, shiny black seed.

Cultivating Woodland Herbs

Before you order any seeds, spawn, or roots to start growing woodland herbs, it's essential to select and, if necessary, prepare an appropriate site. You can grow these herbs in their true habitat in their native woodlands, or you can create areas to mimic those conditions.

Selecting a Site

Unlike most of our garden crops, these herbs allow you to use the shadier parts of your property. All the herbs mentioned earlier grow wild in the understory of deciduous and mixed deciduous and pine forests. They will thrive in areas with 75 to 80 percent shade.

If you're familiar with these woodland herbs, you may have noticed that you will often find them on wooded slopes. All these woodland herbs, including ginseng, bloodroot, goldenseal, and ramps, thrive in well-drained soils. Heavy, bottom clay soils may lead to rotting, disease, and other issues, so it's generally best to avoid them. Where soil is soft and well-drained, you may also find these herbs growing in the bottomlands. Though it may not result in choice herbs, like the wild ginseng preferred in Asian markets, beds may be created and amended to create more suitable soils.

Ginseng, bloodroot, and goldenseal will often grow on north- or east-facing slopes. Southern slopes tend to be drier and sunnier, offering less-than-ideal conditions for these herbs. Ramps may be more tolerant of these areas. Additionally, the slope is less critical at higher elevation areas with consistently cooler temperatures.

You can grow bloodroot and goldenseal in USDA hardiness zone 3 through 8. Ginseng and ramps are generally only successful in zones 3 through 7.

Planting

These herbs may be started from seed, rhizomes, or bulbs. Seeds are usually the most affordable route but often take longer to mature. The seeds of ramps, goldenseal, ginseng, and bloodroot are all fall planted, as are the rhizomes of bloodroot, goldenseal, and ginseng. Ramp bulbs, on the other hand, should be transplanted in later winter or very early spring.

Ramp, goldenseal, ginseng, and bloodroot seed may all take up to eighteen months to germinate. They all require a cold vernalization or a cold period over the winter before germinating. Depending on your plant, location, and conditions, your herbs grown from seed may not reach a good harvestable size for five to ten years. When transplanting rhizomes or bulbs, you may be able to begin harvesting in just three to five years.

When laying out your planting, good circulation and space are essential, especially for ginseng. Leave at least eighteen inches between each plant. One of the reasons ginseng isn't widely cultivated commercially is that when grown in monoculture plantings, ginseng is frequently plagued by disease issues. Making mixed plantings, like of goldenseal and ginseng, can also help.

Plant your ramp bulbs and ginseng, goldenseal, and bloodroot rhizomes about one to two inches deep. Mulch in your newly planted herbs with a good layer of leaf litter. As these are all wild species, you don't need to weed around them, but eliminating competition may help them grow better. You may wish to remove large plants encroaching on your herb's space until you have a well-established colony. Weeding is recommended if you're looking for maximum production in amended beds.

You should not need to water these crops; you typically want to avoid doing so to prevent root rot. If grown in an appropriate habitat, they should get all the water they need. However, you may want to offer some water if you're growing for production in raised or other modified beds. Remember, though, that these herbs prefer moist but not soggy soil.

Harvesting

After you've been through a long wait, you'll finally get to harvest some of your amazing herbs!

In three to ten years after planting, your rhizome pieces or seeds should have grown and spread into a productive patch of herbs. Harvest ginseng, goldenseal, and bloodroot rhizomes in the fall, just after the plant has died back. If you wait too long, it may be hard to identify where the plants are located.

Dig carefully with a garden fork, aiming to keep the fibrous roots and rhizome intact. Large, healthy rhizomes can be transplanted to start new colonies if desired. Avoid harvesting your whole patch; take only a few to ensure you have a continued supply of these at-risk herbs.

Take care when handling bloodroot rhizomes. You may want to use gloves, as bloodroot can cause skin irritation, itching, and redness, especially with prolonged contact.

Harvest your ramps in the spring when their green leaves have unfurled. You can carefully dig the whole plant, eating the bulbs and leaves. However, for more sustainable use, the ramp leaves are just as tasty as the bulbs, and in areas where you're trying to reestablish the plant, harvesting just a single leaf will allow the plant to continue to grow.

All these herbs may be cleaned and dried in a dehydrator for later use. Cutting up the rhizomes will allow them to dry faster and make them easier to use in herbal preparations.

Sourcing Seed, Plants, and Spawn

As all these plants are at risk, getting seeds and roots from ethical sources is important. Do not harvest wild plants to add to your property. Check with local nurseries that offer native plants. A few reliable seed companies, including Johnny's Selected Seeds, Territorial Seeds, Southern Exposure Seed Exchange, and Strictly Medicinal Seeds, now offer some of these for online orders.

References

Authority of the Medical Societies and Colleges. *The Pharmacopoeia of the United States*. Boston: Wells and Lilly, 1820. https://collections.nlm.nih.gov/bookviewer?PID=nlm:nlmuid-2567001R-bk.

Bartlett, Kelsey. "Faculty, Students Spotlight Inequities in Herbal Products Industry." College of Liberal Arts and Human Sciences. Virginia Tech. February 17, 2023. https://liberalarts.vt.edu/news/articles/2023/02/liberalarts-herbal-products-industry.html.

Carlson, Alvar W. "Ginseng: America's Botanical Drug Connection to the Orient." *Economic Botany* 40, no. 2 (spring 1986): 233–49. http://www.jstor.org/stable/4254858.

Cataneo, Emily. "A Plan to Save Appalachia's Wild Ginseng." *Wired*, November 11, 2020. https://www.wired.com/story/a-plan-to-save-appalachias-wild-ginseng/.

Davis, Jeanine M. "Cultivating Native Woodland Botanicals." NC State Extension. Last modified May 18, 2022. https://newcropsorganics.ces.ncsu.edu/herb/cultivating-native-woodland-botanicals/.

Kauffman, Gary. "Plant of the Week: Goldenseal (*Hydrastis canadensis* L.)." US Forest Service. Accessed July 1, 2023. https://www.fs.usda.gov/wildflowers/plant-of-the-week/hydrastis_canadensis.shtml.

Mahr, Susan. "Bloodroot, *Sanguinaria canadensis*." University of Wisconsin–Madison Division of Extension. Accessed July 20, 2023. https://hort.extension.wisc.edu/articles/bloodroot-sanguinaria-canadensis/.

———. "Ramps, *Allium tricoccum*." University of Wisconsin–Madison Division of Extension. Accessed July 20, 2023. https://hort.extension.wisc.edu/articles/ramps-allium-tricoccum/.

Schechter, Alex. "In Appalachia, a Race to Preserve the Practice of Plant Healing." Vox. Last modified May 26, 2022. https://www.vox.com/the-highlight/23023679/appalachia-herbs-gingko-biloba-herbal-supplements.

Downy Mildew–Resistant Basil

⇗ Kathy Martin ⇖

Twenty years ago, when I grew basil in my backyard garden in New England, the plants would be lush and green until the fall frost. Unfortunately, basil is now frequently killed by a newly introduced pathogen, basil downy mildew, as early as midsummer. The good news is that several great downy mildew–resistant (DMR) basil varieties have been developed. Often, nurseries aren't selling these varieties, but hopefully they soon will. I have been growing my own DMR basil plants from seed and will describe my experiences here.

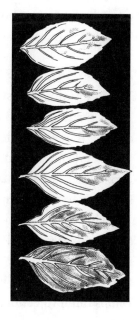

I've been a passionate vegetable gardener for fifty years, starting with 4H in high school and later growing backyard gardens in every home

I have lived in as well as a community garden plot that I've tended for the past fifteen years. My most recent project, Aurelia's Garden, is a two-acre nonprofit farm I help run that grows thousands of pounds of vegetables every year for donation to local food pantries. I'm sure every one of these gardens, even back to the ones I can't remember well, has included basil. Basil is pretty much essential for a vegetable garden.

I used to grow the old-time varieties of classic large-leaf Italian sweet basil, like 'Genovese', 'Italian Large Leaf', and 'Nufar'. I would pick up a few six-packs of the first two varieties at a nursery, or I would grow 'Nufar' myself from seed. They would grow big and vigorously all season. About ten years ago, however (2015, as I remember), my basil plants began to die every year, often by mid-July. I would watch the plants closely for signs of the newly introduced fungus-like pathogen called basil downy mildew and harvest my entire crop immediately when I saw the first symptoms. I'd get a big batch of pesto made, but I'd be left without fresh garden basil for the rest of the season.

What Is Basil Downy Mildew?

The symptoms of basil downy mildew start out with the lower leaves turning yellow, according to Cornell University. This is quickly followed by leaves turning dark brown or black. The leaves curl and wilt, and the undersides develop a grayish-purple fuzz. Observing the fuzzy spores on the underside of the leaves is the key to confirming the presence of downy mildew.

Basil downy mildew is caused by a fungus-like organism (an oomycete) called *Peronospora belbahrii*. When this organism infects basil, the spores germinate and enter basil leaves through pores in the leaves called **stomata**. The pathogen develops thin projections called **hyphae** that penetrate throughout the interior of the leaves and hijack nutrients from the basil plant. Projections exit the plant's stomata and form fuzzy structures that release spores that infect other basil plants.

Basil downy mildew originated in Uganda in the 1930s In 2003 it was discovered in basil in Switzerland. From there, it spread to the United States, first in south Florida in 2007. The next year it was found in field- and greenhouse-grown basil and home gardens across the eastern United States and Canada, as reported by Cornell's College of Agriculture and Life Sciences. In 2008 and 2009, basil downy mildew caused a disaster and devastated commercial basil crops throughout the US East Coast.

Cornell University maintains a monitoring program started in 2009. Reports outside of the United States include Canada, Mexico, Puerto Rico, Costa Rica, Cuba, Argentina, Kenya, South Africa, Turkey, Hungary, the United Kingdom, South Korea, China, Australia, and more. Currently, basil downy mildew occurs in all parts of the world where sweet basil is grown, as reported in the journal *Ecology and Epidemiology*.

Basil downy mildew spreads readily. The pathogen produces abundant spores easily carried by the wind. It is also spread by contaminated seeds and infected seedlings. The organism does not overwinter in cold climates, but each year its spores travel on the wind to the north from warmer areas by midsummer.

Naturally Downy Mildew–Resistant Basils

The sweet basil (*Ocimum basilicum*) that we know as a delicious garden plant is just one species in the genus *Ocimum*. This genus includes more than fifty species of herbs and shrubs from the tropical regions of Asia, Africa, Central America, and South America. While sweet basil is highly targeted by downy mildew, resistance naturally occurs in many wild species.

A study in the journal *Phytopathy* reports that wild basil species such as American basil (*O. americanum*), hoary basil (*O. ×africanum*), camphor basil (*O. kilimanadascharicum*), African basil (*O. gratissimum*), least basil (*O. campechianum*), and tulsi or holy basil (*O. tenuiflorum*) are highly resistant to downy mildew. The close relatives of sweet basil are moderately resistant, including Thai basil (*O. basilicum* var. *thyrsiflorum*), two species called lemon basil (*O. basilicum* var. *citriodorum* and *O. ×citrodorum*), and Greek or spicy bush basil (*O. basilicum* var. *minimum*). Of the species of basil that have been tested and reported on, it is only the cultivars of sweet basil (*O. basilicum*) that are highly susceptible to downy mildew.

An exception is sweet basil cultivar 'Mrihani', the only sweet basil found that is resistant to basil downy mildew. This is an unusual heirloom basil most closely related to Thai basil. 'Mrihani' basil is a traditional herb grown in the East African archipelago of Zanzibar. Its flavor is described as different from either Italian or Thai basil—bright and perfumed with hints of sweet citrus, anise, and fennel. Its leaves are wavy with serrations along their edges.

Growing wild basil is a great way to avoid downy mildew. I often grow Thai basil. It has small, narrow leaves, purple stems, and pink-purple flowers. Its flavor is pungent and spicy with anise and licorice notes. I like to use it in stir-fries and fried rice. I also grow holy basil, which is not a culinary herb but is a pretty plant with purple flowers that attract bumble bees and honeybees.

Development of Resistant Sweet Basil

I was excited when 'Eleonora', the first DMR basil came out. I bought a big packet of seeds. In my experience, I can't say it was much better than the nonresistant varieties. Two other early DMR releases, 'Emma' and 'Everleaf' also have limited resistance.

A big advancement in downy mildew resistance came about five years later in 2019 with the introduction of 'Prospera'. It took over five years for plant scientists at Genesis Seeds Ltd. to develop 'Prospera' because several laboratory steps were needed to produce viable seeds from an interspecies cross between sweet basil and wild hoary basil. Progeny plants of the cross did not produce viable seeds because of the large genetic difference between the two parents. To produce progeny with viable seed, plant scientists used a laboratory procedure called embryo rescue. Hybrids were then produced from the rescued seed, and these now are marketed by Johnny's Selected Seeds and several other seed companies as the variety 'Prospera'. I have grown 'Prospera' for many years. It is a nice vigorous plant with great flavor and has high resistance to basil downy mildew in my garden. Newer releases of 'Prospera' include a series of DMR basil varieties. There is the original tall variety, a couple of compact varieties, and a red basil. I would love to try all these.

'Amazel' is another DMR basil. It is a Proven Winners variety released from the University of Florida that has the same source of resistance as the 'Prospera' varieties. However, its seed is sterile, so it is being sold as cuttings primarily for producing plants for sale in garden centers for home gardens.

Rutgers University Downy Mildew–Resistant Basils

To me, the most exciting development in downy mildew resistance is the series of Rutgers basil varieties. These were introduced a couple of years ago and, in my experience, are amazing. The varieties were developed by "old-fashioned," conventional breeding methods and did not use laboratory manipulation or genetic modification. Rutgers plant scientists spent ten years breeding them.

Conventional plant breeding is a process in which new varieties are developed using natural methods. Parent plants with desirable traits are put together or crossed by natural plant reproduction such that pre-existing traits are mixed and matched to give rise to desirable crops. There are no laboratory steps to rescue fertility or transfer genes. Conventional breeding like this has been used for thousands of years to develop new and better plants.

Basil varieties that are resistant to downy mildew largely do not breed naturally with sweet basil. Crossing them usually produces sterile offspring because the parent varieties are genetically very different. However, Rutgers plant breeders were able to successfully cross the downy mildew–resistant variety called 'Mrihani' with their sweet basil breeding line.

As a result, Rutgers developed four different DMR varieties with the delightful names 'Devotion', 'Obsession', 'Passion', and 'Thunderstruck'. Each has a different growth habit and flavor. The leaf ruffling and serration and the hints of the unusual bright, spicy, and lemony flavor of the 'Mrihani' parent show up in some of the varieties.

I want to emphasize again the conventional breeding approach used to develop the Rutgers varieties. I came across the following comment by Richo Cech, who collected 'Mrihani' seed from Zanzibar. In his seed catalog, Strictly Medicinal Seeds, Cech wrote: "After some time scientists in the US got ahold of this basil and isolated a gene that can be used to confer downy mildew resistance to other culinary basils."

I think it is important to comment that it is a misunderstanding to say that the Rutgers team who made basil crosses using 'Mrihani' basil "isolated a gene." The Rutgers team used only conventional breeding. In contrast, there are other teams of scientists who are working to isolate basil DMR genes. They are using a different basil than 'Mrihani', wild hoary basil, and they have not yet been successful in isolating a gene or doing any directed gene transfers. In fact, no DMR varieties to date (the 'Rutgers' varieties, 'Prospera', and 'Amazel' included) have been made by isolating genes or by gene transfer methods. They are all made by crosses followed by selection for resistance.

Rating the Rutgers Varieties

At Aurelia's Garden we grew a sixty-foot-long row of all four Rutgers varieties this year. This row totaled about 250 plants, about sixty of each variety. A group of about eight of our farm volunteers tasted them in mid-October. Our findings are included here:

'Rutgers Obsession DMR': The growth of this plant is a little more compact than the other Rutgers selections. It has dark green, thick, flat, glossy leaves. The leaves have an Italian aroma and flavor with slightly earthy, spicy notes. Some of our taste testers described the flavor as an earthy, warm spice taste like cloves, and maybe a hint of tack room leather. It is sweet, basily, and just right for pesto. It was a favorite for many of us, the mildest of the four. It is also a plus that it is the only one of the four that is highly resistant to Fusarium wilt disease.

'Rutgers Devotion DMR': These plants have uniform, upright growth, growing to about two feet tall. They have large, slightly ruffled, serrated leaves that are medium green with a lightly sweet and spicy aroma. We found it to be sweet at first with a sharp aftertaste, the sweetest of the four varieties with a very good herbal taste. However, some testers did not like it and described it as flavorless with a sharp, aggressive aftertaste.

'Rutgers Thunderstruck DMR': This variety ranks highest of the Rutgers basils for downy mildew resistance. The plants are very high yielding. They are medium sized with fast, upright growth. The leaves are lovely, ruffled with a bright green color like the 'Mrihani' parent. Some of us found this to be a wonderful minty-tasting basil, sharp and herbal with lemon overtones. For some, it was a favorite because it was different. However, a group of us did not like this variety, describing it as too strong with an unpleasant aftertaste. They felt the flavor would be too strong for a classic sweet basil pesto.

'Rutgers Passion DMR': This is a beautiful basil. The leaves are large and slightly cupped and rank the highest of the Rutgers basils for classic Italian sweet basil flavor. We found it to be very nice: slightly sweet, spicy, and savory.

Cornell has been studying DMR basil since 2010, and in 2018, they added the Rutgers varieties to their trials. A Cornell report from the Long Island Horticultural Research and Extension Center from twelve different field sites ranked the basils on a scale of 1 to 10, with 10 being. In order of best flavor, they rated 'Passion' (6.8 for taste, 8.2 for marketability, 7.6 for appearance), 'Prospera' (6.5, 6.6, 7.5), 'Thunderstruck' (6.4, 5.2, 5.9), 'Amazel' (6.3, 8.6, 9.1), 'Obsession' (6.2, 6.6, 6.8), and then 'Devotion' (3.7, 2.2, 2.3).

How Does Basil Resist Downy Mildew?

The basil plant's immune system becomes active when it tries to fight downy mildew. This includes genes detecting the pathogen, transducing signals, and responding to the infection. Many plant receptors are always on the lookout for pathogens. Once a pathogen is detected, signaling cascades become active. Signaling leads to responses by the plant, including preventing further infection, inhibiting pathogen reproduction, blocking the activity of pathogen molecules, and breaking down the pathogen itself.

What do the new resistant basil varieties do to resist downy mildew? Researchers who developed 'Prospera' are trying to answer this question. So far, Rutgers researchers have mapped the region of genes that confer resistance and shown that this region includes a major resistance gene plus two other three genes that work together. Plant scientists at Genesis Seeds have shown that the Prospera DMR has a single duplicate dominant resistant gene (Pb1). The two teams of researchers continue to work to identify individual genes and functions in the hopes of being able to use directed genetic modification in the future. An exciting article was recently published by Johnny's Selected Seeds that connected several basil DMR researchers, including the Genesis Seeds breeder of 'Prospera' DMR, Dr. Arnon Brand. This article describes the connection and friendship between the 'Prospera' and Rutgers groups and cites the optimistic view that solutions are in the pipeline for continued development of vigorous basil downy mildew resistance.

We now have more than a dozen DMR basil varieties available to growers and home gardeners. Why do we need so many? The first part of the answer is that they all have different tastes and appearances. But a second part is that there is concern the pathogen could evolve to overcome host resistance. Pathogens are always evolving. If we have many basil varieties, each with a different mechanism of resistance, we will have the others to fall back on if one becomes ineffective against the disease.

Where Can You Get Seeds?

Unfortunately, I haven't yet seen DMR plants available in garden centers near me. My friends who grow plants that they buy at garden centers have ended up with nonresistant varieties that succumb rapidly to downy mildew. This coming year, I will grow plants from seed for them. Very soon I expect to see 'Amazel', the Proven Winners variety, marketed in my area. But Proven Winners products can be pricy. To me, it makes sense to grow your own plants from seed if you can.

Rutgers DMR basil seeds are available to home gardeners from several online sources, though 'Obsession' and 'Devotion' are easiest to find. 'Obsession' and 'Devotion' are sold by Johnny's Selected Seeds, High Mowing Organic Seeds, Whitwam Organics, Harris Seeds, Osborne Quality Seeds, Seedway, Gardener's Supply Company, Stokes Seeds, and several other online vendors. 'Passion' is currently at Harris Seeds. 'Thunderstruck' can be ordered from Stokes Seeds, Ball Seed, and Condor Seed. Seed for four of the varieties are grown and distributed for home gardens by KBC Specialty Seeds. VDF Specialty Seeds produces bulk seed for commercial basil growers. Though I have not yet seen the Rutgers basil seeds in garden centers at the time of this writing, I expect they will be there soon.

Growing DMR Basil from Seed

Sweet basil is a relatively easy herb to grow from seed. It's a lot easier than slow-growing herbs like thyme and rosemary. I plant basil at the same time as my tomato seeds, late March, which is six to eight weeks before my last spring frost. In areas with a winter temperature that falls below freezing, basil seeds should be started indoors and grown under lights before transplanting out to the garden.

Sow seeds about ¼ inch deep and thin seedlings to about ½ inch apart. I like to start basil in 4 × 4-inch pots. Germination requires 5 to 10 days at 65 to 70 degrees Fahrenheit (18–21°C). All basil varieties are subject to damping off, a fungal disease triggered by moisture. To prevent damping off, start basil plants in fresh seed-starting mix using clean tools and new or disinfected pots. (To disinfect pots, soak them in a 1:600 dilution of bleach in water for 20 minutes.) Avoid overwatering and overcrowding seedlings. Use a fan for air movement around the seedlings. When the seedlings get their second set of leaves, transplant each to a single pot or cell of a 6-pack and continue to grow under lights or in a warm greenhouse. Transplant out to the garden after all chance of frost is gone and the nights are about 50 degrees Fahrenheit (10°C). These methods are the same as I use for any type of basil, whether it is Thai basil, holy basil, or sweet basil.

When the plants begin to mature, keep the flower stalks picked off. Though the bees love them, the plants will senesce and die if they are allowed to put their energy reserves into flower and seed production. (Wild basils do not need to be deadheaded.) Sweet basil plants will benefit from regular harvesting. When plants reach about 15 inches in height, clip off branches, leaving about 8 inches of height to the plant.

It's October as I write this, and my crop of this year's basil will probably die in the next week when Boston temperatures are predicted to drop well into the forties at night. It's been a good year for basil. It has enjoyed the abundant rain we've had, and it's not as dependent as other tropical plants, like tomatoes and squashes, on heat and sun, which we have been lacking in New England this year. At my farm, we have covered our basil with row cover to try to get another week's harvest from it. I look forward to trying a new set of basil varieties next year and seeing what our ever-changing weather will bring us.

Resources

Ben-Naim, Yariv, Lidan Falach, and Yigal Cohen. "Transfer of Downy Mildew Resistance from Wild Basil (*Occimum americanum*) to Sweet Basil (*O. basilicum*)." *Phytopathology* 108, no. 1 (2018): 114–23. doi:10.1094/PHYTO-06-17-0207-R.

Chec, Richo. "Basil, Mrihani (*Ocimum basilicum*) Seeds, Organic." Stricly Medicinal Seeds. Accessed October 17, 2023. https://strictly medicinalseeds.com/product/basil-mrihani-ocimum-basilicum -seeds-organic/.

Cohen, Yigal, Yariv Ben Naim, Lidan Falach, and Avia E. Rubin. "Epidemiology of Basil Downy Mildew." *Phytopathology* 107, no. 10 (2017): 1149–60. https://doi.org/10.1094/PHYTO-01-17-0017-FI.

Cornell Vegetables. "Basil Downy Mildew." Cornell University. Last modified March 2023. https://www.vegetables.cornell.edu/pest -management/disease-factsheets/basil-downy-mildew/.

Long Island Horticultural Research and Extension Center. "Basil Downy Mildew." Cornell University. Accessed October 17, 2023. https:// blogs.cornell.edu/livegpath/research/basil-downy-mildew/.

Pyne, Robert, et al. "A First Linkage Map and Downy Mildew Resistance QTL Discovery for Sweet Basil (*Ocimum basilicum*) Facilitated by Double Digestion Restriction Site Associated DNA Sequencing (ddRADseq)." *PLOS One* 12, no. 9 (September 18, 2017): e0184319. https://journals.plos.org/plosone/article /file?id=10.1371/journal.pone.0184319&type=printable.

Rutgers University. "Four New Rutgers Sweet Basil Varieties Are Available to Home Gardeners." Rutgers Today. June 24, 2019. https://www.rutgers.edu/news/four-new-rutgers-sweet-basil -varieties-are-available-home-gardeners.

Under-Cover Gardening: Extending Your Growing Season through Winter

⤗ Monica Crosson ⤖

As August wanes and the sun begins to drop along the horizon,
there is a melancholy that settles deep
within me, for I know that summer
is ending and darker days are closing
in. I am one who relishes the raucous
growth of spring in the garden and
lounges under the soothing mellow
light of summer. There is something
about the earth at her pinnacle that
feeds my soul and enlightens my
senses—the hum of insects and the
scent of honeysuckle, the taste of
fresh tomatoes and flashes of sun
across the pond. I require less sleep,
rising to the early morning calls of
the grosbeak and not resting until
well after dark when the frogs have
grown weary of their croaking.

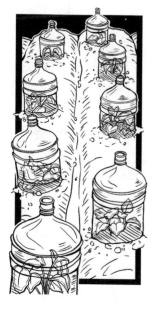

Autumn is forced upon me, and I reluctantly accept her dark mantle, reminding me that there is beauty in decay. Leaves turn to shades of crimson and ochre, and an ethereal mist fills the river valley as the temperature cools. Winter arrives on lonely gusts that test my patience and have me sometimes questioning its promises of spring's return.

But there is a spark of summer's fruitfulness that I hold on to during the darkest days of the year. For tucked safely in cold frames and in containers cozied safely under house eaves, leafy greens and bright violas are a reminder that, indeed, life still lingers in winter's frosty grip. Fresh herbs and vegetables are a welcome treat throughout the winter season, and with a little forethought, anyone can extend the growing season, no matter where they live.

Extending Your Growing Season

The end of the summer typically means the end of fresh herbs and vegetables for those of us who keep a garden in colder regions. But with a little ingenuity, hardy vegetables, herbs, and even flowers can be grown long into the darkest months.

Before you start making plans for the tomato, squash, and peppers that flourished all summer long, let's take a look at a few basics to make winter gardening easier. The first thing to remember to be a successful winter gardener is to not try to grow your garden as you would in the summer. Look for cold-hardy varieties of plants that do well in your plant hardiness zone. If you're not sure what yours is, you can access a hardiness zone map online or on page 215 or talk to someone at your local university extension office.

Next, we have to start preparing for our winter garden while the sun is still high. Most seeds need to be planted anywhere from late July until late August. I suggest purchasing seeds for your winter garden when you purchase your summer garden seeds and just setting them aside. Plant starts for some winter gardening favorites (such as cabbage) are available from local gardening centers around August.

You may be wondering what kind of plants you can grow for winter. Once again, that will depend on the region you live in and your garden setup. If you live in a warm region (zones 9 to 11), winter gardening can be a very productive time. Peas, lettuce, brassicas, kale, and carrots grow easily with the cooler temperatures. Large, heated greenhouses can also easily extend gardens for those in cooler regions. When I have my greenhouse going, I can extend my tomato production until late November. For those of us who live in regions with mild or wet winters (zones 7 to 8), sometimes just an added layer of straw is enough to protect herbs, leafy greens, and root vegetables all winter long. But for many regions, winter temperatures can drop well below freezing, requiring a little extra care to keep the garden producing.

Gardening Under Cover

Because not everyone has the space, time, or money to set up a large greenhouse for their winter gardens, these easy solutions make it possible for anyone to grow leafy greens, herbs, and root vegetables all season long.

Polytunnels: Working the same as a greenhouse, polytunnels use the sun's rays to hold the heat and provide a controlled environment for your plants. They are easy to set up and can surprisingly hold a lot of weight (for those who get a lot of snow). They are basically a series of plastic, metal, or wooden hoops used as a frame covered with polythene. They can be as large as a greenhouse or as simple as a low row cover.

Cold Frames: These easy-to-make shelters are basically a wooden box with a transparent lid (like an old window) on a hinge, which plants can be grown in all winter long. If you have zero carpentry skills, they can also be made by surrounding your bed with straw bales or bricks and using polythene stapled to a wood frame as a lid.

Cloches: Popular throughout the nineteenth century, cloches are bell-shaped glass covers used to protect tender plants threatened by frost. Today, glass cloches can be expensive, but plastic ones are available online or at garden centers. They are both inexpensive and reusable. You may also consider making them out of your discarded plastic milk, soda, or juice containers or out of large glass jars. Just place your cloche over a single plant or small group of plants during times of extreme cold.

Winter Garden Fare

Did you know that some vegetables taste better after a good cold snap? Carrots, beets, cabbage, turnips, and kale are sweeter in the winter. Cool-weather crops like root vegetables and leafy greens need that chill to turn starch into sugar and give them their wonderfully sweet taste. Who knows, maybe after you sample winter beets or brussels sprouts, they may become a new family favorite. Here is a list of vegetables you may want to try in your winter garden:

Arugula (**Eruca vesicaria**): Winter-harvested arugula has a mild, nutty flavor. Direct sow in August for greens all winter long. Try 'Roquette' or 'Speedy'. Zones 3–11.

Beets (**Beta vulgaris**): Direct sow in late July for a winter harvest. Try 'Winterkeeper' or 'Red Ace'. Zones 2–11.

Broccoli (**Brassica oleracea** *var.* **italica**): Sow indoors in July and transplant in your garden in August. Try 'Belstar' or 'Apollo'. Zones 2–11.

Brussels Sprouts (**Brassica oleracea** *var.* **gemmifera**): Sow indoors in early June for late July transplant in your garden. Try 'Franklin' or 'Igor'. Zones 3–9.

Cabbage (**Brassica oleracea** *var.* **capitata**): Sow indoors in early June and transplant in the garden in early August. Try 'Late Flat Dutch' or 'Tundra F1'. Zones 3–10.

Carrots (**Daucus carota**): Sow directly in your garden in late July to early August. Try 'Napoli' or 'Nantes'. Zones 3–10.

Kale (**Brassica oleracea** *var.* **sabellica**): Direct sow in mid-July for late fall and winter harvests. Try 'Dwarf Siberian' or 'Red Russian'. Zones 4–10.

Kohlrabi (**Brassica oleracea** *var.* **gongylodes**): Growing sweeter after the first frost, direct sow from late July to mid-August to enjoy until spring. Try 'Superschmelz'.

Leeks (**Allium porrum**): Direct sow between March and June for winter harvest. Try 'Giant Musselburgh' or 'Bleu de Solaise'. Zones 5–9.

Lettuce (**Lactuca sativa**): Direct sow through September for lettuce all winter long. Try 'Winter Density' or 'Cimmaron'. Zones 3–10.

Mâche (**Valerianella locusta**): Also called "corn salad," mâche is a delicate, refreshing green that can be directly sown between August and October to enjoy throughout the winter. Try small-seeded mâche for winter growing. Zones 4–9.

Parsnips (**Pastinaca sativa**): Sweeter after the first frost, sow in late July. Try 'Gladiator F1' or 'White Gem'. Zones 2–9.

Radishes (**Raphanus sativus**): Direct sow in August through September. Try 'China Rose' or daikon. Zones 2–11.

Spinach (**Spinacia oleracea**): Direct sow until the end of October for vitamin-packed greens all winter long. Try 'Giant Winter' or 'Sunangel'. Zones 2–9.

Turnips (**Brassica rapa *subsp.* rapa**): Direct sow in August to enjoy throughout the winter. Try hakurei or 'Purple Top White Globe'. Zones 2–9.

Potatoes in a Can

Potato (*Solanum tuberosum*) tubers are a great cool-weather crop and grow wonderfully in mounds, bags, or containers. It makes sense that they do well as a late fall to early spring vegetable. A quick-growing solution for even the smallest yard is using a garbage can. In late August to early September, drill several drainage holes in a 10-to-20-gallon garbage can and place it in an area that gets full sun. Fill with approximately 6 inches of compost. Leave a few organic potatoes out on the counter to sprout (a process known as **chitting**), and place 3 to 6 in the soil. Add 3 to 4 inches of composted soil on top and water in. For every 10 inches of growth, add 3 to 4 more inches of compost, remembering not to cover the leaves with soil. Do this until the garbage can is full and your leafy stems are growing above the rim of the can. After potato plants bloom, they will begin to wilt, and you need to stop watering. Once the greens are completely withered, you can dig up your potatoes and enjoy. Full maturity is reached in 70 to 120 days. Try fast-growing varieties like 'Cliff Kidney' and 'Swift' in zones 3 to 10.

Easy Winter Container Gardens

You don't have to have a sprawling landscape and yards of row cover to enjoy winter gardening. If you have a porch, balcony, or deck space with southern exposure, you can extend your growing season by using containers. To protect them further from chilly winds and colder temperatures, tuck them close to walls, fences, shrubs, or doorways. Pairing easy-care flowers and herbs with greens such as kale, lettuce, and cabbages makes for a lovely addition to your outdoor spaces, and you'll have easy access from the kitchen on those deary days one would rather not venture any farther than the back door. When temperatures drop below freezing, you may want to consider using cloches.

Soil requirements for winter containers are different from those for the typical growing season, especially if you live in a rainy climate (like the Pacific Northwest). Soil can become oversaturated, resulting in root rot or mold. Make sure to use a good-draining potting soil or a "soilless" mix. You can buy a soilless mix in any garden center or make it yourself using the following recipe.

ᴁ Soilless Potting Mix

There are many DIY mixes to fit your garden's nutritional needs, but this all-purpose blend is great for winter containers.

You will need:

    2 gallons sphagnum peat moss

    2 gallons fine compost

    1 gallon perlite

    2 tablespoons lime

    ½ cup organic fertilizer (5-5-5 mix)

Mix the components together and use the blend in your containers, beds, or boxes for winter planting.

Recommended Plants for Winter Container Gardens

The following is a selection of flowers, herbs, and vegetables perfect for your winter containers.

Winter-Hardy Flowers for Containers

- Creeping Jenny, *Lysimachia nummularia* (zones 4–9)
- Coral bells, *Heuchera sanguinea* (zones 4–9)
- Cyclamen, *Cyclamen persicum* (zones 4–8)
- Dutch crocus, *Crocus vernus* (zones 3–8)
- Hellebore, *Helleborus ×hybridus* (zones 6–9)
- Heather, *Calluna vulgaris* (zones 5–8)
- Indian chrysanthemum, *Dendranthema indicum* (zones 5–9)
- Ivy, *Hedera helix* (zones 4–10)
- Ornamental cabbage, *Brassica oleracea* (zones 2–11)
- Pansies, *Viola ×wittrockiana* (zones 6–10)
- Violas, *Viola* spp. (zones 6–10)
- Winter aconite, *Eranthis hyemalis* (zones 4–7)
- Winter creeper, *Euonymus fortunei* (zones 5–9)

Winter-Hardy Vegetables for Containers

- Beets, *Beta vulgaris* (zones 2–11)
- Cabbage, *Brassica oleracea* var. *capitata* (zones 3–10)
- Carrots, *Daucus carota* (zones 3–10)
- Kale, *Brassica oleracea* var. *sabellica* (zones 4–10)

- Lettuce, *Lactuca sativa* (zones 3–10)
- Radishes, *Raphanus sativus* (zones 2–11)

Winter-Hardy Herbs for Containers
- Chives, *Allium schoenoprasum* (zones 3–10)
- Greek oregano, *Origanum vulgare* (zones 5–9)
- Mint, *Mentha* spp. (zones 3–8)
- Parsley, *Petroselinum crispum* (zones 2–11)
- Sorrel, *Rumex* spp. (zones 5–9)
- Thyme, *Thymus vulgaris* (zones 5–9)

⤜ *Wintertide Kitchen Container*

This lovely container gives a pop of color to your porch while also providing commonly used herbs and vegetables to brighten your winter meals.

You will need:

    2 'Red Russian' kale

    2 red-tinged loose-leaf lettuce

    1 curly parsley

    2–3 'Cool Wave Raspberry' pansies

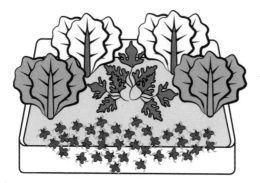

In a large container (24 inches across or more), plant 'Red Russian' kale to the back, followed by the lettuce on each side of the parsley situated in the middle, and lovely cascading pansies in the front.

Winter is a time of contemplation and hope. And those vegetables, herbs, and flowers that manage to keep producing long into winter keep that spark of summer alive. I enjoy being able to have fresh vegetables all season long, and I hope this sparks you to carry on a little bit of summer's fruitfulness through the winter.

The Wonders and Benefits of Volunteer Plants in Perennial and Annual Herb Gardening

⤞ Geoffrey Edwards ⤝

In the realm of gardening, there is beauty in allowing nature to take the lead. By embracing the concept of volunteer plants, gardeners can witness the wonders that unfold as various greens spring up naturally from seeds dispersed by the hands of nature. This article delves into the enchantment and advantages of cultivating volunteer plants in both perennial and annual herb gardens, highlighting their ability to enhance biodiversity, provide medicinal benefits, and offer a bountiful harvest throughout the seasons.

Volunteers

Sometimes, the most valuable contributions to our herb gardens arrive

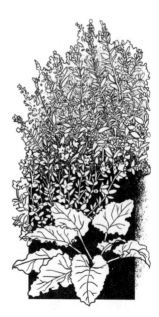

uninvited. Despite our intentional efforts in creating and cultivating gardens, certain herbs find their way as volunteers.

Wineberry, *Rubus phoenicolasius*, was among the first welcome volunteers that I can remember making an appearance in the corner of the garden. I was intrigued by what I perceived on the stems to be small red thorns but, on close examination, found to be red hairs. These unexpected additions bring not only beauty but also a wealth of edible, nutritious, and medicinal properties found in the raspberry-like berries and leaves.

Over the years, I noticed when blankets of **greater periwinkle** (*Vinca major*) flowers adorn the ground beneath the crepe myrtle tree growing on one gently sloped corner of the garden, it serves as a message from nature. Spring is ushering us to officially shed our winter lethargy and embrace the growing season. These volunteer plants not only add visual appeal with their beautiful pale violet flowers but also signify the awakening of a vibrant and productive ecosystem.

Within the garden, the inclusion of creeping aromatic herbs such as **thyme** (*Thymus vulgaris*), **hyssop** (*Hyssopus officinalis*), **marjoram** (*Origanum majorana*), and **oregano** (*Origanum vulgare*) along the pathway creates a sensory experience for barefoot walking meditations, tai chi, and qigong practices. The morning dew and essential oils released from the herbs gently massage the soles of the feet as you walk across the stone path, providing therapeutic benefits for achy bones and joints and an immune system boost.

Foraging Favorites

Among the various growing beds, the forage bed stands out as this gardener's favorite. With minimal intervention, this bed thrives through the efforts of volunteer plants reseed-ing themselves and the presence of perennials I have planted. Burdock, wild violet, plantain, Indian strawberry, dandelion, lamb's-quarters, alfalfa, wineberry, yellow dock, amaranth, and pawpaw densely populate this space. It may not be the most aesthetically pleasing area, but it offers an abundance of wild greens that can be harvested almost year-round, provid-ing an accessible, invaluable resource for fresh and healthy meals.

I was always interested in using the garden to encourage and cultivate plants whose parts can all be utilized. Volun-teer plants like **lamb's-quarters** (*Chenopodium album*), which provide edible seeds that can be dried, toasted, and ground into flour or cereal similar to quinoa, fulfills this purpose. Ad-ditionally, collecting the seeds in the fall and sprouting them throughout the winter months ensures a continued supply of nutritionally dense sprouts packed with chlorophyll. The leaves are delicious when prepared as one would spinach and other tender leafy greens. The roots are also a powerhouse, great for assisting the bowels to eliminate waste from the body when there is stagnation within that bodily system.

Hands down, my favorite plant with multiple beneficial parts is **mulberry** (*Morus* spp.). Different parts of the plant are used for different therapeutic purposes, and they are often com-bined with other herbs to create specific formulas tailored to the individual's condition. Mulberry holds a special place for me because it is one of the first volunteers that I became familiar with when I was a student of acupuncture and Chinese herbal medicine. I was amazed that one plant could possess this much potential. Mulberry leaves, known as *sang ye* in Chinese, and the fruit, *sang shen*, have long been used in traditional Chinese medicine (TCM) for their potential to treat respiratory illnesses, diabetes, and high blood pressure. Mulberry twigs and roots have also been used in traditional Chinese medicine for various purposes. Mulberry twigs, known as *sang zhi*, are often used to address conditions such as joint pain, stiffness, and muscle spasms, as noted in *Chinese Herbal Medicine: Materia Medica*. They are believed to have anti-inflammatory properties and are commonly used in formulas for arthritis, rheumatism, and similar ailments. Mulberry roots, known as *sang bai pi*, are primarily used as a diuretic and expectorant. They are often used to address respiratory conditions such as coughs with thick phlegm, lung congestion, and excessive fluid retention. Mulberry root is also believed to have cooling properties and is used to alleviate heat-related symptoms, including fever and thirst. Overall, the mulberry tree stands as a testament to nature's healing potential, as its different parts provide a range of medicinal benefits.

Common **evening primrose** (*Oenothera biennis*), another delightful volunteer, finds its way annually to borders, edges, and neglected areas of the garden. Evening primrose attracts beneficial predatory insects like the spined stilt bug (*Jalysus wickhami* Van Duzee), which aids in reducing the populations of aphids and hornworms, thereby maintaining a balanced ecosystem. Though the seed oil is prized for being rich in many health-improving benefits, the evening primrose in my garden is left to grow just to the point after flowering. Then I deadhead the spent blooms and make sure to later prune close to ground level.

Plants like **pokeweed** (*Phytolacca americana*) intrigue us with their dual nature of being both medicinal and fatally toxic. Every spring when harvesting the young pokeweed greens, I get a glimpse into the challenges faced by Indigenous herbalists and foragers throughout history. These plants remind us of the reverence and apprenticeship required to wield such powerful knowledge. Understanding the correct stage of development, the appropriate plant parts to harvest, and the necessary preparation methods are vital to ensuring safety and harnessing their potential benefits. Besides, pokeweed is simply a sight to behold, its beauty captivating when mature, with blood-red colored stems and dark purple berries contrasting its green lanceolate leaves.

Not only do perennial plants require less maintenance than annual plants, but they are also a great consideration to help restore soil health.

Volunteer TCM Remedies

Perennial herb gardening offers a world of wonders, even during the off-season. The simplicity of winter colors and textures in nature allows us to appreciate the distinct characteristics of plants. As we explore the garden and woods, we discover the hidden treasures of herbs that provide both beauty and medicinal benefits. From the edible flowers of rose of Sharon to cinnamon vine bulbils, these perennial plants offer a wealth of possibilities. Join me as we pivot on our journey through the fascinating world of perennial herb gardening and discover the joys of cultivating your own natural remedies.

During winter, the **rose of Sharon** (*Hibiscus syriacus*) stands out with its distinct colors and textures. While its green foliage may be gone, the plant's branches, bark, and stems catch the eye. This perennial herb not only adds beauty to your garden but also offers medicinal and culinary uses. The leaves and flowers are edible and can be used as garnish in dishes and salads. Additionally, hummingbirds, butterflies, and bees are attracted to the flowers, adding life and vibrancy to your garden. The plant's seeds, a favorite of small birds during winter, can also be consumed. Moreover, the leaves and flowers contain mucilage, which can soothe sore throats and provide relief for burns and hot skin conditions.

Cinnamon vine (*Dioscorea polystachya*), also known as *shan yao* in TCM, is a captivating perennial herb that also offers both nutritional and medicinal value. Now considered invasive in many states in the United States, cinnamon vine has a long history of use in Chinese medicine. I love the way the vines delicately climb on the trellis in their container. Cinnamon vine is one of the volunteers that popped up in the garden, so I decided to observe ways I could work with and not against it, since the tubers were such a challenge to dig out. Because these are non-native plants that propagate easily, I build beds around them and trellis with bamboo to make pruning easy when the bulbils grow. Each year I use sculpture wire and wood to create interesting shapes for the vine to grow on, which always adds an artistic element to the garden. Not only is cinnamon vine fun to make art with, but this versatile root vegetable is rich in dietary fiber, which aids in digestion, promotes a healthy gut, and enhances overall vitality. Cinnamon vine yams are believed to nourish the spleen, stomach, and lungs, and the plant is often used to boost energy and regulate blood sugar levels, shares nutrition researcher Paul Pitchford in *Healing with Whole Foods*.

Burdock (*Arctium lappa*), with its beautiful flowers and abundance in the wild, is a rewarding addition to any herb garden. In my garden it thrives as a volunteer and as a planted herb. This biennial herb offers various benefits, from its edible roots rich in minerals to its seeds used for clearing heat in the body. The roots can be sautéed or added to soups, providing a diuretic effect and supporting the kidneys and liver in eliminating toxins naturally, notes food educator Andrew Sterman in *Welcoming Food*. Meanwhile, the seeds, known as *niu bang zi* in TCM, serve as a natural remedy for sore throats, fevers, and other symptoms associated with heat in the body. As we face increased pathogens, having burdock on hand becomes invaluable, especially for making soothing teas. Adding burdock root to our natural home remedies list is a wise choice, particularly during the detoxifying spring season.

Baikal skullcap (*Scutellaria baicalensis*), known as *huang qin* in TCM, is known as a reliable herbal of choice for clearing heat in the body and lowering blood pressure. This perennial herb proves particularly useful for treating conditions such as fevers, colds, infections, irritability, and respiratory conditions such as cough with profuse yellow phlegm, according to *Chinese Herbal Medicine*. It may also be used for digestive issues such as diarrhea and liver problems and to support the immune system. Oftentimes when working near the bed of the baikal skullcap, I observe the delicate dance of the small bees and other pollinators in the hooded sapphire blue flowers. This highlights the plant's significance not only as a pollinator attractor but also as a natural remedy, and it emphasizes the importance of incorporating perennials into our yards.

Similarly, **balloon flowers** (*Platycodon grandiflorus*), also known as *jie geng* in TCM, are invaluable for respiratory health. Just before the flower opens, balloon flowers look just like a sea of blue-violet hot-air balloons about to take flight from the garden. As I sit with the balloon flowers, I am reminded of how the canopy of lungs fills with air similarly. However, it's the other end of the plant where the true benefits are found. The roots of this perennial herb are used in TCM to promote lung health, reduce inflammation, and alleviate coughs, wheezing, and sore throats, making it an essential ingredient in herbal formulas, as shared in *Chinese Herbal Medicine*. By strategically placing these plants throughout the yard, we ensure a steady supply of medicine for years to come in our family.

———

Perennial herb gardening is a captivating journey that reveals the wonders of nature's medicine cabinet. The wonders and benefits of volunteer plants in perennial and annual herb gardening are truly marvelous. From the visual delight they bring to the garden to the medicinal properties they possess, these volunteers have immensely enriched my gardening experience. From the beauty and versatility of the rose of Sharon to the nutritional benefits of cinnamon vine and the diverse medicinal properties of burdock, baikal skullcap, and balloon flowers, these plants offer an array of possibilities. By embracing their presence and allowing nature to take its course, we can cultivate a thriving ecosystem that provides beauty, sustenance, and a connection to the natural world. Embrace the joys of perennial herb gardening, and the next time you spot a volunteer plant, try to get proper identification so you can welcome it as a gift from nature and witness the magic it may bring to your garden.

Resources

Bensky, Dan, Steven Clavey, and Erich Stöger. *Chinese Herbal Medicine: Materia Medica*. 3rd ed. Seattle, WA: Eastland Press, 2004. Pages 131–32, 429–30, and 763–64.

Pitchford, Paul. *Healing with Whole Foods: Asian Traditions and Modern Nutrition*. Berkeley, CA: North Atlantic Books, 2002. Pages 342 and 550.

Sterman, Andrew. *Welcoming Food*. Bk. 1, *Energetics of Food and Healing*. Ann Cecil-Sterman, 2020. Pages 145 and 166.

Create an Herb Garden Paradise

↠ James Kambos ↞

My grandparents, James and Katina, were Greek immigrants. They eventually settled in a small Ohio town located in the foothills of Appalachia. There, they opened a tavern and diner in the picturesque and historic downtown. Along with their four children, including my mother, Mary, they lived in an apartment located above the business. My grandfather came home one day and told my grandmother that he didn't want his children being raised over a tavern. He then made an important announcement: he had bought a house.

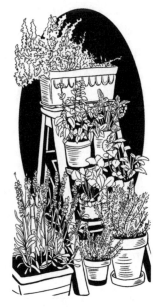

It was a large, rambling, white two-story house. Located at the edge of the business district, it was just a block away from my grandparents' business. Steps led up from the street to a large concrete porch that wrapped around two sides of the house. The covered porch provided much-needed shade, a great relief on a humid southern Ohio summer afternoon. The only yard was a grassy hillside that rose steeply to the street behind the house.

Even though the size of the yard was limited and the lot was steep and oddly shaped, it lit a creative spark inside my grandmother. To her, it was a blank canvas. It gave her the creative outlet she yearned for. She quickly turned a cramped finger-shaped residential lot into an oasis of herbs and flowers. It stopped traffic. Passersby would slow down to catch a glimpse of this colorful speck of earth. The arbor covering the stairs leading from the sidewalk was hugged by a pink climbing rose. Pots of herbs important to Greek cooking were everywhere—mint, dill, oregano, and basil. A tender potted jasmine that had to be carried indoors every fall took center stage. Perennials and annuals of every description covered the hillside with a mix of color. Visitors were greeted by color and fragrance.

One warm summer afternoon, the mail carrier paused as he made his deliveries and remarked, "Coming here is like stepping into paradise."

It's time to create your own garden of paradise, no matter how large or how small.

Creating Your Herb Garden Paradise

It may sound strange, but your garden design begins indoors. That's right, good garden design begins with the style you feel most comfortable living with inside—contemporary, country, traditional, and so on. Next, your home's architectural style will most likely determine your garden's design elements. For example, a contemporary home with modern architectural style would probably have a garden with clean straight lines. Paths would likely be concrete, and plantings would be spread out.

A country-style interior may have a cottage-type architectural exterior. Fences might be a picket style, covered with climbing roses, and the yard might have curved planting beds, planted more thickly. Paths might consist of stepping stones.

And a traditional-style home inside and out might use brick for paths or for edging a plant border. Plantings would probably be a little more formal.

Also, colors you love to live with inside are usually echoed outside in a well-planned garden. Don't forget, the color of your exterior doors and shutters is another good way to decide on the colors of herbs and flowers that you wish to feature in your garden.

Designing your herb garden ahead of time will help elevate your herb garden from just a garden to a paradise.

Over time, your style and tastes will probably change. Don't be afraid to let those changes show in your herb and flower garden. Eventually, my grandmother moved to a one-floor ranch-style home on a suburban street. She was still passionate about gardening, but the style of her new home was reflected in her garden. She began to incorporate rock gardens, each with a theme. And with more space, she now included shrubs, trees, and even a vegetable garden in her garden plot.

Style and Planting Tips

There are no wrong or right garden styles, herbs, or flowers that you should select for your garden. However, there are ways to plan and plant your garden to give it the most charm and eye appeal.

Let's begin with the shape of your beds and borders, a subject I touched on earlier.

If your home is a mid-century ranch or a new contemporary design, your beds would probably complement your home's style and be straight and uncluttered. Paths that are concrete or gravel would likely look the best. And among the herbs and flowers, plant a few ornamental grasses. They're easy to maintain, and their foliage will add softness to the straight lines of the borders and paths.

A country style or rustic design such as a cabin would blend perfectly with the informal look of curved beds. A trellis or arbor covered with an old-fashion climbing rose would lend charm. Allowing low-growing culinary herbs such as thyme to spill onto a garden path would also add to the charm of a rustic setting. In this type of space, paths consisting of stepping stones or pine needles would be the perfect final touch.

Traditional homes would most likely have outdoor spaces that look a bit more formal. Materials such as stone or brick would be perfect if used for patios or paths. Edging herb and flower beds with boxwood also adds to the traditional feel.

Gardening Suggestions

Regardless of your herb garden's style, the following suggestions will enhance any garden setting and make your garden environmentally friendly.

Leave Room for Pollinators

Any herb garden should help our beneficial birds and insects. Herbalists of long ago knew that. They always included a few of these herbs to help the birds, bees, and butterflies. The plants I've selected are easy to grow, dependable, and non-invasive. Try a few of these: black-eyed Susan, blazing star, coneflower, and woolly betony.

Plant in Odd Numbers

If space permits, plant herbs in clumps of threes. One is fine, but three of one variety gives dramatic impact.

Plant with a Theme

Any herb garden gains added interest when a bed or a border is planted with a theme. One example is color. A bed planted with only silver- or gray-colored foliage is beautiful. Or try a bed planted with only one scent, such as lemon or mint. Herbs with these scents will delight the nose and lift the spirit.

Raised Beds

Some of the greatest herbalists I've met incorporated raised beds into their garden design. Raised beds are easy to care for and each raised bed could easily have its own theme. Also, raised beds can be separated by paths consisting of gravel, pine needles, stone, or simply grass. Any of these options would heighten the visual appeal.

The Power of Pots

Planting herbs and flowers in pots is a huge asset to any herb garden. They'll go a long way in helping you create that herb garden showplace you're dreaming about. Pots and planters can help you highlight certain plants, add color, create visual interest, and help mark off an entry point leading to a different area of your herb garden. Pots also allow you to observe the growth habits of an herb. This way you can see if you like a particular herb or flower before you plant it directly into the garden. And don't forget, a pot will allow you to grow tender herbs and flowers that you can't winter over directly in the garden. That's how my grandmother kept her prized jasmine year-round in Ohio. It was brought inside every fall, then moved back to the terrace every May.

To give your herb garden paradise a natural feel,
try adding a few stones or pieces of wood
in interesting shapes.

Let's take a look at pot materials and styles. Pots and planters come in a huge variety of materials, styles, and sizes. Materials include plastic, metal, stoneware, wood, and traditional clay. Styles can be anything from a fancy urn to a humble clay pot. No matter what your scheme, it'll be perfect. For example, one of my favorites is an antique metal sap bucket from New England. It only cost a couple of dollars. I added some drainage holes, and right now it has a place of honor on the deck in my herb garden, filled with a fern and impatiens.

When selecting pots for your herb garden, remember, clay and stoneware pots are more porous and may require more frequent watering. Plastic and metal pots retain moister longer.

Other Garden Features

To make your herb garden paradise complete, consider adding finishing touches such as benches, statuary, or a tasteful shed. When it comes to benches, place them where they'll really be used. Stop and consider the view and the natural light at different times of the day.

For statuary, consider pieces that blend with your landscape. And bigger isn't always better. Frequently, a small statue can have great impact when nestled amid the foliage of herbs or ferns. It creates a charming niche and allows a visitor to your garden to feel as if they've made a discovery.

If you need a shed, think about constructing one that will echo the architecture of your home. For added charm, include a path leading to its door, a window, and a window box overflowing with herbs or flowers of your choice.

Making It Fertile with African Natural Farming

ᾥ Mason Olonade ᾥ

I have been fascinated with the concept of building healthy black soil outside of the traditional composting method after reading an article on farming practices in Liberia and Sierra Leone in the journal *Human Ecology*. The natural farming styles Korean natural farming, Japanese natural farming, zero-input Indian natural farming, and the new style I document with *Jigijigi: Africulture Podcast*, African natural farming, all follow a core principle in different languages that translates to "do as nature does." Nature doesn't build mounds or use bins, turning them every so often, balancing the browns and greens. Trees grow, leaves grow, leaves fall, trees grow.

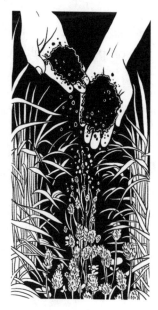

So how were and are the Loma and Mende peoples building the *porleilei*, or "black-black" soils? How are they making it fertile? They produce fires for cooking, making palm oil and potash, and spread those ashes, char, and wastes from production over their fields. However, the most interesting soil-building strategy is their communal living and waste management. The end product of living life their way creates immensely fertile soils that go down, in one area, six feet deep, share university researchers in an article in *Frontiers in Ecology and the Environment*.

Waste from harvests, food production, weeds from around the compounds, worn thatch roofs, tools and brooms that have reached the end of their lives, insect wings and carcasses, old clothes, bones, shells, guts and scales, and human and animal manures are placed in an area called *tulupole* (dumpsite soil) in Loma or *kawei* (dumpsite) in Mende. Charcoal from charcoal production and old fires, along with ash, is spread over the dumpsite. As this process is repeated over the years, the micropores within the charcoal become perfused with the juice of decomposed organic matter and microbiota.

Building Porleilei for Home Gardens

With some modifications, this approach of building porleilei is accessible to us too! I invite you to join me in creating porleilei with the paint can biochar method and black soldier flies.

Making Biochar

Obtain a small paint can from a local hardware store. Punch several holes into the lid. Stuff the can full with organic matter and seal it. I use the shed branches of the river birch (*Betula nigra*) and red maple (*Acer rubrum*) in my front yard. Larger branches from storms are used to fuel the fire. Build a fire that can burn for two hours. This paint can **retort** you have built, stuffed, and sealed can now be tossed into the fire. It will begin to steam, and then wood gases will be distilled out of the wood, catching fire and speeding up the charring process. When piles of brush are burned on the farmlands in Sierra Leone and Liberia, they are set on fire from the top. When the flames burn down instead of up, the bottom of the pile is starved of oxygen and pyrolysis occurs, creating charcoal. After two hours, we have recreated their process.

Now in order to transform this charcoal into biochar, we have to charge it, but what do we charge it with? With anything that can be decomposed or is ready for recomposition.

Anaerobic Fermentation and Black Soldier Flies

When I sealed a bucket of overripe okra (*Abelmoschus esculentus*) in five gallons of water and opened it up a month later, it reeked of horse manure. I didn't expect this and delved deep to understand this anaerobic composting. I was corrected, finding out that composting is decomposition in the presence of oxygen. What I performed was **anaerobic fermentation**. Said more poetically, by sealing that container, life at its most ancient, the archaea and eukaryotes, devoured the okra and turned it into five gallons of divine fertilizer. Best of all, it was entirely passive! No turning or protecting, no fences or traps, just life going on as it always has. However, because it is more likely we will not set up the structures to harvest and use the methane gas that is produced, we will recruit black soldier flies (*Hermetia illucens*) instead.

Last spring, I set out a bucket of springtime kitchen scraps to attract the black soldier flies. Days went by and my lid started resting on top of rinds—nothing had changed! Then the fruit flies came. Going out to the area on the deck that my wife and I call the "nursery" became a real drag. Flies everywhere! My wife didn't go outside. I tried to appease her by telling her that the fruit flies' gut microbiome contains *Acetobacter*, and if they land in some old wine, we can have our own vinegar. I kind of succeeded; she was grossed out and mentally moved on.

A week later I looked out of the window of the hospital room my son was born in and a voice spoke to me, "The flies will now arrive." Several sleep-deprived days later, I checked the bins and I was startled. Movement! Squishing, churning, funky, grotesque movement! The voice spoke truth! The black soldier flies had arrived in great quantities and pushed out all the other flies and gnat populations.

With my larvae in place, I added the charcoal I made to the buckets. This is where we improvise within the structure of our folk science by adding somewhere around a 2:1 ratio of black soldier fly bucket contents to charcoal. A different way to do this is to get another bucket, pour half of the black soldier fly bucket into the new bucket, and add charcoal to the new bucket. Don't worry about filling up your new bucket. Once in the bucket, and especially throughout the growing seasons, the larva frass juices permeate every pore of the charcoal, making a rich, nutrient dense fertilizer and soil amendment. When the frost kills my larvae, their carcasses further contribute, with their exoskeletons and the chitin therein amending the soil even more. This year the tulupole is complete. Our journey to building porleilei has begun.

Farming with the Ancestors

As we create our porleilei, we must consider what we are also doing: Creating the conditions for more life. Creating structures for more life to exist within our soils, within our farms, within our communities—this is how we make it fertile. Creating more life in this realm and in realms beyond us. How do we create spaces for the ancestors to grow alongside us, as the Kuranko and Kissi farmers of Guinea do?

Tombondu are long-abandoned villages that are defined by their fertile soils and productive plantings. These settlements were once-infertile savannah that was settled, farmed, and left fallow. The fallow period resulted in a food forest instead of savannah. This area has been cultivated by the ancestors and, after careful consideration and propitiation, is cultivated by the people.

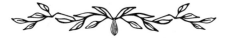

If you live in a neighborhood surrounded by deer, seed sweet clover into your lawn in the winter, and come spring, you'll never mow again!

We must create tombondu in our growing spaces. How do we figure out how to get places where spirit moves in and grows? We create a plot for our ancestors, for them to grow alongside us, in conversation, showing us how to grow what is truly necessary.

In the book *Test Your Soil with Plants*, John Beeby recommends leaving a plot of land within your land wild to gauge the nutrient profile of your soils. Each weed that grows tends to have a relationship with certain nutrients in a deficiency or surplus. By restoring the soil to normal—meaning, by bringing reciprocity and balance to the soils—we rid ourselves of the weeds. As you may be independently familiar with, Korean natural farming discusses using the weeds around us to make fertilizer to grow the plants we want to grow, because those plants growing well in our environment have within them, by virtue of their growth, what is needed to grow healthy and strong in that environment.

With these methods in mind, I'll state that, when welcomed, the ancestors are growing what is literally required to grow healthy black soils, for us to make fertile. By creating tombondu for them, they grow plants for the tulupole for us, and in turn we create porleilei. These weeds can be anaerobically fermented, charred, or partially rotted and fed to black soldier fly larvae to render them into fertilizer. Incorporating these techniques will produce profound and remarkable changes in the health of your soil, your crops, and within you! However, you may lose track of time. Try to think of it as a small sacrifice, an exchange for connecting with your land.

Spirit of the Farm

Those familiar with permaculture understand the concept of ecological succession. Our farm in Charlotte also understands that concept really well and is constantly working to turn itself back into the woodlands that border it to the north.

One morning within the farm, tired of weeding tree saplings, I spread my arms out in embrace, faced the woods and said, "Spirit of the Forest, I understand you wanting to turn this land back into woods. I want you to understand our intentions with this land. We aren't farming here in spite of you, in defiance of you, or in ignorance of you. It is my intention to create within the minds of the youth here an appreciation of you through growing food for their families and neighbors on your land. You may not know, but when the construction begins for the co-op, they will cut through even more of you, reducing you by half.

"Spirit of the Forest, please use your energies of growth toward our crops, to build our health so we can advocate for your preservation and conservation. Can you work with us, please?"

The next Saturday I entered the farm gates. As usual, I surveyed the rows and the soil, checking for mushrooms and caterpillars, when I was interrupted with a quiet but looming "Okay."

With a confused expression, I snapped my head up toward the forest. I understood!

Subsequently, as I unlock the gates, I offer this prayer before I enter the farm, which you can try as well. Please adapt it to suit your cosmology.

> *Spirit of Nature, Spirit of the Farm, Spirit of the Forest*
> *Spirit of Nature, Spirit of the Farm, Spirit of the Forest*
> *Thank you for another day*
> *Thank you for welcoming me and bringing me here safely*
> *Thank you for giving me the opportunity to cultivate the health, wealth, and spirit of the soil, of the crops, and of the people in the community*
> *Keep my eyes open to issues I need to address, plants that need care, and all that I need to see*
> *Asante Sana, Medase Pa, Modupe O! (Thank you, thank you, thank you!)*
> *Asè, asè, asè (Amen equivalent)*

Then I enter the farm. Invariably, things begin jumping out at me, good things, like pine warblers and goldfinches dance-battling for echinacea seeds (*Echinacea angustifolia*), and bad things—well, good things that I have no immediate use for—like corn smut (*Ustilago maydis*) spreading uphill from the downhill infected corn plot (*Zea mays*). Either way, it fits our schema, it is a sign of life, and we create spaces for more and more life.

Holistic and Community Applications

After two years of volunteering at this farm, I took the opportunity to become the Farm Manager of the Three Sisters Farm and Seeds for Change Program for the West Boulevard Neighborhood Coalition here in Charlotte, NC. The farm was founded as a request from the community to have local access to fresh healthy foods. This area has been deprived of a full-service grocery store for over forty years. After years of unsuccessful attempts to woo larger chains through subsidy, the community decided to do it for themselves. The farm was started as a proof-of-concept, proving the moral and financial demand was present for these goods and services. The next step is currently being taken to build the West Boulevard Neighborhood Cooperative Grocery Store. So far we've obtained considerable support from local and congressional representation.

The Seeds for Change Program is where we employ youths aged fourteen to eighteen in the community to grow food (and themselves) organically. From June until Thanksgiving, I work with the young men and women in that community to do just that. Now that I was in charge, I was so excited to share all that I have shared with you, dear reader, with the youth, strategies on "making it fertile" and other historical approaches of African natural farming. I couldn't wait for the school year to end. We were going to all test out my theories! The spirits of nature, the farm, and the forest had other plans.

I found myself becoming a therapist instead. One afternoon, I pulled my phone from my pocket and pressed the green phone key. The mother of one of the youths, Demetrius, was calling. "Mr. Mason, Demetrius will not be at the farm today. Apparently, he's been skipping school, I want you to keep an eye on him when he gets back. Make sure he ain't out there playing with his friends."

Demetrius was fifteen. He told me the reason why he was at the farm was to develop more discipline to become a better father for his daughter. She was three.

His mother continued, but customers began lining up and other boys started to arrive, so I said, "Yes, ma'am, I understand. I'll keep you posted. Talk to you soon!"

Twenty minutes later, Demetrius arrived, immediately shed his jacket, and got straight to work. This was highly unusual. Normally, he headed toward the storage container, ate two bags of chips, drank one and a half bottles of water, changed his shoes, and meandered down the hill to the entrance to ask me what to do. Something was very wrong.

I told everyone else what to do and walked up the hill to Demetrius, who was watering the cover crops opposite the corn stalks.

"Demetrius, what's this I hear about you skipping school?"

"Man! See wh—" I shook my head and motioned to pump the brakes, and he restarted. "Sorry, Mr. Mason, aight, so boom, I sit in the front of the class, and everyone around me is making noise during attendance, so I can't hear my name being called, and they mark me absent!"

Plausible deniability was granted to Demetrius, as one of the other boys at the farm confirmed the teachers' behavior at their high school.

"Look, Demetrius, because of the choices you have made, your mother is worried about your capacity to make decisions. Can you see that?"

He nodded.

"So you need to apologize to her, and this is how you do it. First, you tell her 'this is why it looks like this,' without blaming anyone. Second, 'this is how I contributed to it looking like this.' Third, 'this is what I've done to make sure it doesn't happen again.' This is your template. I'm not going to tell you what to say, but saying that your way will go a long way with her."

He got back to work and I looked at the corn. "Demetrius, based on this interaction with your mom, would you say you are frustrated?"

Through clenched teeth, he responded, "Absolutely."

"Come with me."

We walked out of the farm to the storage container. I grabbed a machete and we walked back to the corn plot. We had just got a fancy electric hedge trimmer, but why bother using it when I've got fifteen-year-old boys with energy to burn?

"Demetrius, I am going to give you catharsis. Do you know what that means?"

"I've heard that word before, but I forgot it."

"I want you to take this machete and chop all this corn down. Direct all your frustrations into chopping these stalks smaller and smaller. You'll know when you are finished. But! We can't just be destructive—we must organize our emotions once we've released them. So you're going to get a rake and rake up these stalks back into the rows. Then you'll spread that crimson clover over the rows and this whole area. That crimson clover is then going to grow up and through your chopped stalks, making fertilizer from your emotions for next year. Do you understand?"

He nodded, and I placed the machete in his hands. He floated over to the corn plot, fashioned his undershirt into a headband, and got to work. I knelt close by, picking cowpea pods (*Vigna unguiculata*), and then I had an idea. Just as I was turning around to share it with him, he said, "Mr. Mason, can I keep this?"

"I was just about to say you should keep one of the stalks to remember this!"

On the last day of the program, after all the customers left and the tools were placed and locked away, I exit-interviewed the boys who stuck with me through the growing season. I asked them each to go to their favorite spot on the farm. One of the boys, Mohammed, stayed put right by the trunk of my car.

"Why are we standing here, Mohammed?"

"Because this is the spot where I get paid."

I met Demetrius standing in the middle of the corn plot, rows even, straight, pristine, with crimson clover creeping through the chopped stalks.

"Why are we standing here, Demetrius?"

"Because this is the spot where I solved my anger issues."

———

I started *Jigijigi* to investigate African natural farming and to share strategies for how to build healthy soils and healthy souls. It appears that the plan of these spirits was to show me that it works. Rather than a strict protocol for how to grow a crop,

I hope you've found inspiration for how to grow your green thumb with African natural farming. The work that the youth, the community, the spirits, and I performed with this framework has resulted in full blackberry canes (*Rubus allegheniensis*) eight feet tall, gladiolus flowers (*Gladiolus* ×*hortulanus*) over six feet tall, a 250 percent increase in honey production, and more youth working—making it fertile.

Resources

Beeby, John. *Test Your Soil with Plants!* 2nd ed. Willits, CA: Ecology Action of the Midpeninsula, 2013.

Fairhead, J., and M. Leach. "Amazonian Dark Earths in Africa?" In *Amazonian Dark Earths: Wim Sombroek's Vision*, edited by William I. Woods, Wenceslau G. Teixeira, Johannes Lehmann, Christoph Steiner, Antoinette WinklerPrins, and Lilian Rebellato, 265–78. New York: Springer Science, 2009.

Frausin, Victoria, James Angus Fraser, Woulay Narmah, Morrison K. Lahai, Thomas R. A. Winnebah, James Fairhead, and Melissa Leach. "'God Made the Soil, but We Made It Fertile': Gender, Knowledge, and Practice in the Formation and Use of African Dark Earths in Liberia and Sierra Leone." *Human Ecology* 42, no. 5 (2014): 695–710. doi:10.1007/s10745-014-9686-0.

Olonade, Mason. 2021. "Smelling Funk to Power." *Jigijigi: Africulture Podcast*, May 1. Podcast, 12:40. https://africulturepodcast.com /smelling-funk-to-power/.

Solomon, Dawit, Johannes Lehmann, James A. Fraser, Melissa Leach, Kojo Amanor, Victoria Frausin, Søren M. Kristianson, Dominique Millimouno, and James Fairhead. "Indigenous African Soil Enrichment as a Climate-Smart Sustainable Agriculture Alternative." *Frontiers in Ecology and the Environment* 14, no. 2 (2016): 71–76. doi:10.1002/fee.1226.

Cooking

Pizza for the Seasons

≫ Sara Mellas ≪

From fresh basil leaves scattered atop Neapolitan-style margherita pizzas to glass shaker bottles of dried oregano sitting on tables at pizza shops, herbs are a common ingredient in the world's most popular food. But beyond basil and oregano, there is a garden's worth of other herbs that can be used to make creatively topped, delicious pizzas.

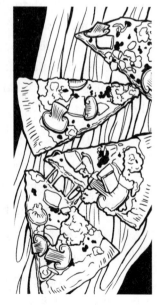

While dried herbs are readily available and many fresh herbs can be grown and purchased year-round, there is something special about using certain herbs to enhance seasonal flavor profiles. And what better way to enjoy the flavors each season has to offer than with homemade pizza?

Whether you're a *pizzaiolo* or brand new to making pizza, read on to learn the best practices for baking pizza at home.

The Dough

Most pizza dough is a simple combination of flour, water, olive oil, yeast, salt, and a pinch of sugar. However, how it's kneaded, risen, and baked, as well as the baker's altitude and the day's weather, will effect significant variations in the final result.

If you're a regular at baking bread and working with yeast, you'll likely enjoy making homemade pizza dough. A stand mixer with a dough hook attachment is not entirely necessary, but it is incredibly helpful for obtaining the correct gluten structure and overall success.

If you prefer to have your pizza sooner rather than later, store-bought dough is a perfectly fine option! Most grocery stores sell balls of freshly kneaded dough in the bakery or prepared foods section. There are also several brands of commercially prepared dough made specifically for home ovens that are sold in the dairy aisle. Many pizza shops will allow customers to buy unbaked dough directly from them to take home—just ask!

⇏ Pizza Dough

1⅓ cups warm water

1 packet (¼ ounce) instant yeast (2 teaspoons)

1½ teaspoons sugar

1 tablespoon olive oil

¾ teaspoon salt

3½ cups (425 grams) bread flour or all-purpose flour, plus more as needed

1. Lightly oil a large mixing bowl and set aside.
2. Place the water, yeast, sugar, oil, and salt in the bowl of a stand mixer fitted with a dough hook attachment. Turn the mixer to low.
3. Begin slowly adding the flour. Once it's incorporated into the wet ingredients, turn the mixer to medium.* Allow the mixer to knead the dough until it is smooth and elastic, about 8 to 10 minutes. The dough should be quite tacky, but not sticky. If it's too wet, add a few tablespoons of flour to achieve the desired texture.
4. Collect the dough from the mixer and shape it into a ball. Transfer the ball to the oiled mixing bowl and cover it with plastic wrap or a clean kitchen towel. Set the bowl in a warm place and let the dough rise for 1½ hours, or until it's doubled in volume.
5. Gently punch down the dough and reshape it into a ball. It's now ready to be rolled for pizza.

Baking Pizza in a Home Oven

Baking pizza at home differs from baking pizza in a restaurant kitchen, and the results, while still delicious, are simply not the same. This is primarily due to the temperature of commercial pizza ovens, which heat to upward of 1,000°F. The initial blast of heat opens the crumb structure of the crust and bakes it rapidly, creating a crispy, blistered exterior and a chewy, airy interior.

---

* If you do not own a stand mixer, this dough can be kneaded by hand. It may take up to 15 minutes until it reaches the desired smoothness and elasticity.

While this may not be safely attainable in a home oven, there are ways to approximate it and still end up with crave-worthy pizzas.

For starters, if you plan on making pizza at home somewhat regularly, a pizza stone is an inexpensive and worthwhile investment. The stone helps conduct heat more effectively than a standard pan. However, a dark-colored metal baking sheet will do fine.

Place the stone or pan on the lowest rack of your oven and keep it there while the oven preheats. Preheat your oven to as hot as it will go—for most home ovens, this is 475 to 500°F. Once the oven is at temperature, allow it to stay there for at least 30 minutes, keeping the door closed, before baking your pizza. This helps replicate the aforementioned blast of heat that occurs in commercial ovens.

If using homemade or a store-bought ball of pizza dough, roll it as thinly as is possible without tearing. If the dough is resisting, let it rest for a few minutes, then roll again. This allows the gluten to relax and become easier to work with.

If using commercially prepared store-bought dough (i.e., the kind sold in a tube), do not preheat your oven to as hot as it will go. These doughs are specifically intended for home ovens and have added ingredients that accelerate baking and browning. Therefore, it is best to simply follow the baking instructions on the package.

Once your pizza dough is rolled and topped, transferring it to the oven can be a bit tricky. If you own a pizza peel, carefully slide it under the assembled pizza, place it directly on the hot pizza stone in the oven, and then swiftly slide it out. Alternately, you can roll and assemble your pizza on top of a sheet of parchment paper, slide the parchment and pizza onto a baking sheet or large cutting board, and then slide it off the baking sheet onto the hot pizza stone. Either way, move slowly and mindfully, as unbaked pizza is a bit precarious and the oven is very hot!

While the pizza bakes, do not open the oven door for the first 10 minutes, preferably waiting until the 11- or 12-minute mark to see if it is done. Be just as careful removing the pizza from the oven as you were putting it in. Allow the pizza to cool for at least 5 minutes, then slice with a wheel cutter or sharp knife.

Herbs by Season

Most herbs are quite durable plants, sustaining across months and overlapping seasons. We're also fortunate to live in a time when modern growing practices make fresh herbs available all year long. That said, some herbs peak in the warmer seasons, while others thrive in the cooler seasons, and their flavors pair best with either spring and summer or fall and winter harvests.

Spring and Summer: Basil, chives, chamomile, cilantro, dill, fennel, lavender, marjoram, mint, oregano, parsley, summer savory, thyme

Fall and Winter: Bay leaf, chervil, ginger, anise, mint, rosemary, sage, tarragon, thyme, winter savory

Let yourself be inspired by seasonal produce and have fun experimenting with different combinations of vegetables, cheeses, and herbs. Purists may say differently, but there are no rules to what you can and can't put on pizza! Spring, summer, fall, and winter—there is a pizza for every season, and the following recipes will get you started. *Buon appetito!*

Spinach and Feta Pizza with Lemon-Garlic Oil and Dill

Inspired by Greek spanakopita, this springtime pizza is brushed with bright lemon-and-garlic-infused olive oil and covered with baby spinach, tangy feta, and zippy dill. It can be served as a light dinner or topped with a sunny-side-up egg and eaten for brunch.

You will need:

½ cup extra-virgin olive oil

2 cloves garlic, grated

Zest of 1 lemon

¼ teaspoon dried oregano

14-to-16-ounce ball pizza dough

1½ cups fresh baby spinach leaves, loosely packed

½–¾ cup shredded low-moisture mozzarella cheese

½ cup feta cheese crumbles

1 to 2 sprigs fresh dill, roughly chopped

1 to 2 medium eggs (optional)

1. Pour the olive oil into a resealable container and stir in the garlic, lemon zest, and oregano. Seal the container and let it sit at room temperature for at least 15 minutes.

2. Set a pizza stone or pan on the bottom rack of the oven. Preheat the oven to 475°F. Once at temperature, allow it to stay closed for at least 20 minutes before baking the pizza.

3. Turn the pizza dough onto a sheet of floured parchment and roll it as thinly as possible, approximately ¼-inch thick. Brush the dough with a coat of the infused olive oil. Arrange half the spinach leaves on top, then

sprinkle evenly with the shredded mozzarella. Top with the remaining spinach leaves. Scatter the feta cheese and chopped dill on top.

4. Gently crack 1 or 2 eggs on top of the pizza (optional).

5. Carefully transfer the pizza to the hot pizza stone or pan. Bake for 11–14 minutes, until the crust is golden brown and the cheese is fully melted. If you added eggs, the whites should be opaque but the yolks still runny. Remove the pizza from the oven.

6. Allow it to cool for 5–10 minutes. Drizzle with a bit more infused olive oil, if desired, then slice and serve.

➳ Summer Farmers' Market Basil Pesto Pizza

When the summer markets and farmstands are overflowing with juicy tomatoes, sweet corn, and lush basil, pizza is a delicious and convenient means of enjoying the bounty. A modest blend of Italian cheese and fresh mozzarella allows the produce to shine atop the crust, and a handful of arugula leaves adds a peppery finish.

If it's simply too hot outside to turn on the oven, this pizza can be baked on the grill!

You will need:

14-to-16-ounce ball pizza dough

⅓ cup basil pesto (homemade or store-bought)

⅓ cup shredded Italian blend cheese (or low-moisture, part-skim mozzarella)

4 to 6 ounces fresh mozzarella, torn

½ cup halved cherry tomatoes

1 ear fresh corn kernels

1 cup loosely packed arugula leaves

1. Set a pizza stone or pan on the bottom rack of the oven. Preheat the oven to 475°F. Once at temperature, allow it to stay closed for at least 20 minutes before baking the pizza.

2. Turn the pizza dough onto a sheet of floured parchment and roll it as thinly as possible, approximately ¼-inch thick. Spread an even layer of basil pesto and sprinkle evenly with the shredded cheese. Arrange the torn mozzarella on top, then scatter with the halved cherry tomatoes and corn kernels.

3. Carefully transfer the pizza to the hot pizza stone or pan. Bake for 11–14 minutes, until the crust is golden brown and the cheese is fully melted. Remove from the oven.

4. Allow to cool for 5–10 minutes. Top the pizza with fresh arugula leaves, then slice and serve.

☙ *Butternut Squash, Apple, and Bacon Pizza with Thyme Honey*
With fall comes shorter days, long-awaited harvests, and celebrations. This comforting pizza showcases thin slices of butternut squash and tart apples alongside creamy goat cheese and savory bits of bacon. A sweet drizzle of thyme-infused honey adds a delicate layer of irresistible flavor to every bite.

Make a double or triple batch of thyme-infused honey to use in other recipes or to sweeten tea. Allow it to cool completely, and then store it in an airtight jar at room temperature.

You will need:

¼ cup local honey

3 sprigs fresh thyme, divided

½ small butternut squash

1 tart red apple (like 'Pink Lady', 'Honeycrisp', or 'Fuji')

14-to-16-ounce ball pizza dough

3 slices bacon, cooked and roughly chopped

⅓ cup crumbled goat cheese

Neutral cooking oil

Coarse sea salt

1. Set a pizza stone or pan on the bottom rack of the oven. Preheat the oven to 475°F. Once at temperature, allow it to stay closed for at least 20 minutes before baking the pizza.

2. Place the honey and 2 sprigs of thyme in a small saucepan and set it over medium heat. Allow the honey to come to a simmer. Once simmering, turn down the heat to medium-low, and continuing simmering for 1–2 minutes longer, until the thyme is fragrant. Remove the pan from the heat and set aside.

3. Peel the butternut squash and remove the seedy innards. Slice crosswise as thin as possible, so that the slices appear almost shaved. Core the apple, leaving the skin on. Slice into ⅛-inch slices.

4. Turn the pizza dough onto a sheet of floured parchment and roll it as thinly as possible, approximately ¼-inch thick. Brush the dough with a thin coat of thyme-infused honey. Arrange the squash and apple slices on top. Scatter with the chopped bacon and goat cheese. Sprinkle the leaves from the remaining sprig of thyme over the pizza. Gently brush or spray the toppings with a thin coat of oil.

5. Carefully transfer the pizza to the hot pizza stone or pan. Bake for 11–14 minutes, until the crust is golden brown and the squash appears slightly caramelized. Remove the pizza from the oven.

6. Allow it to cool for 5–10 minutes. Drizzle with thyme-infused honey and sprinkle liberally with sea salt. Slice and serve.

⫸ Mushroom, Caramelized Onion, and Rosemary Pizza

Savory-sweet and buttery, caramelized onions serve as the base for this wintery pizza. Topped with earthy mushrooms, rosemary, and a mix of mild Italian cheeses, it can be served as a delicious appetizer at a holiday gathering or as a comforting meal on a cold night.

The caramelized onions can be prepared as indicated in step 3 up to 5 days in advance. Keep them refrigerated in an airtight container until use.

You will need:

1 medium yellow onion

1 cup cremini or baby bella mushrooms

2 sprigs fresh rosemary

3 tablespoons salted butter

14-to-16-ounce ball pizza dough

1½ cups shredded Italian blend cheese (or a mix of mozzarella, provolone, parmesan, and asiago)

1. Set a pizza stone or pan on the bottom rack of the oven. Preheat the oven to 475°F. Once at temperature, allow it to stay closed for at least 20 minutes before baking the pizza.

2. Peel the onion and cut it in half from top to bottom. Slice each half into very thin, scant ¼-inch strips. Slice the mushrooms. Roughly chop the rosemary leaves, discarding the stems.

3. Set an extra-large sauté pan over medium heat and add the butter. Once melted, add the sliced onion and stir to coat. Cook until the strips are lightly golden, then lower the heat to medium-low. Continue cooking, stirring occasionally, until the onions are extremely soft and caramel brown. This may take up to 20 minutes. Remove the pan from the heat and set aside.

4. Turn the pizza dough onto a sheet of floured parchment and roll it as thinly as possible, approximately ¼-inch thick. Scatter the caramelized onions evenly over the dough, then arrange the sliced mushrooms on top. Sprinkle evenly with the shredded cheese, followed by the chopped fresh rosemary.

5. Carefully transfer the pizza to the hot pizza stone or pan. Bake for 11–14 minutes, until the crust is golden brown and the cheese is fully melted. Remove the pizza from the oven.

6. Allow it to cool for 5–10 minutes, then slice and serve.

Embrace a Meatless Monday

≈ Laurel Woodward ≈

I've always had a vegetable garden. Gardening is in my blood. I grew up with a family vegetable garden in Arizona, a tradition I held tight to and managed to pass to my husband and children. Now we all have the gardening bug. My daughter and oldest son love to work with the earth as much as I do. My middle child is a collector of plants and seeds that he brings home and gifts to me, while my youngest keeps order by weeding, trimming, and mowing.

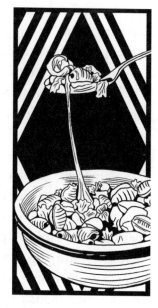

Our family vegetable garden encompasses half an acre of organic pastureland that we converted into gardening space. For us, gardening is a joy, and tending it is a therapeutic mind-body activity that exercises muscles and builds strength while reducing stress and expanding feelings of well-being. Spending time working the earth and helping a plant grow is a balm for the soul. The activity encourages the mind to be present. It expands awareness to fill the world with color, and as we glimpse the awe of nature, it kindles a deeply felt sense of wonder. In that instant, life becomes brighter as the heart grows light.

The vegetable garden also provides us with a source of healthy food and grants the exploration of a diversity of vegetables not found in most grocery stores. For example, I have 'Brandywine' and 'Cherokee Purple' tomatoes, 'Amish Pie' pumpkins, 'Bright Lights' swiss chard, and eggplants, which markets in my area do not stock. From the first sprigs of spinach and peas in the spring to the corn and squash crops of fall, we grow it all.

I take special pride in knowing exactly what went into growing each crop and that the only hands it passed through were my own. The vegetables did not travel any distance to make it to my table, and since the garden is organic, I know for certain that they are free of toxins, pesticides, and herbicides. The corn is not a GMO variety, and the tomatoes are heirloom varieties that taste delicious. As the season progresses, the biggest problem becomes what to do with the surplus. Too much zucchini? Try a recipe for zucchini muffins or zucchini cake. Have you tried zucchini lasagna? Having a seasonal abundance of a vegetable sparks an exploration that rewards the gardener-cook with a repertoire of healthy, easy-to-make, tasty dishes that they can expand upon each season. There is something incredibly satisfying about nurturing a crop until you have an abundant supply just outside your door that you can cook up into nutritious, satisfying meals to nourish your family.

Vegetables are good for you! They provide nutrients, vitamins, and compounds necessary for good health. According to the USDA's latest health models, half of each plate of food we eat should be composed of fruits and vegetables. If dietary needs allow, not only does eating more vegetables improve health and help make you feel great, but a diet low in meat and high in produce is also good for the environment.

Animal agriculture is taking a toll on the earth. Raising animals for slaughter uses up land and water, driving farmers to clear-cut our valuable forests. It also takes a lot of grain to feed the animals—two to five times more per calorie than if we just ate the grain ourselves. In fact, it is estimated that one third of all crop land is used to feed livestock instead of people, writes Bernard Marr for *Forbes*. The sheer numbers of the animals themselves generate nearly the same amount of greenhouse gas emissions as those from global transportation, reports the Humane Society International. Even as stark as these facts are, today's demand for meat is growing.

The Power of Meatless Meals

But there is hope. A new study published in *PLoS Climate* found that if we curb our meat usage, we could gain the ability to stabilize the greenhouse gas levels and in turn gain more time to wean our dependency on fossil fuels. It is within our power to be the change and make a difference. If each of us dedicates one or two days a week to eating meatless meals, we can heal the earth.

I am lucky that my family loves vegetables. We eat a lot of meals made from our homegrown produce. Even though one kid cringes at the sight of a mushroom and another hates olives, there are many vegetable dishes that have come to be family favorites. I'm not talking rabbit food, though I do love a good salad. I mean delicious, comforting, stick-to-your-ribs meals that fill you up for hours.

One of my favorite ways to prepare a zucchini, eggplant, or butternut squash is to simply roast it in the oven. Cut the vegetable into slices, drizzle the slices with olive oil, and bake at 400 degrees Fahrenheit until tender. Then season with salt and pepper to taste, and voilà, you have delicious food brimming with nutrients. Turn this side dish into to a meal by adding pasta, rice, beans, or potatoes and topping it with cheese, and suddenly you've got a delicious, good-for-you meal that is both hearty and satisfying.

Here are a few recipes to help you on your quest:

Fresh Corn Fritters
2 cups fresh corn kernels

¼ cup diced red pepper

2 tablespoons cornmeal

1 teaspoon sugar

¼ teaspoon baking powder

1 teaspoon salt

2 eggs, separated

4 tablespoons olive oil

2 cups salad greens

1½ cups shredded cheddar cheese

Preheat your oven to 350°F. In a mixing bowl, stir together the corn, pepper, cornmeal, sugar, baking powder, salt, and egg yolks.

In a separate bowl, whip the egg whites until stiff peaks form. Fold the egg whites into the corn mixture. Then heat 2 tablespoons olive oil in a skillet. Working in batches, scoop up ¼ cup batter and drop on the skillet. Cook for 2 minutes, then flip, flattening slightly with the spatula. Cook until the fritters are golden brown.

To serve, divide the greens among 6 plates. Place 2 hot fritters on the pile of greens and top with a generous amount of cheese for a deliciously satisfying meatless meal. Makes 6 servings, or about 12 small fritters.

ᚱ Greens and Fresh Pea Frittata

8 large eggs

⅓ cup whole milk

Generous, heaping ½ cup queso fresco cheese

Scant ½ cup freshly grated parmesan cheese

2 tablespoons olive oil

1 cup chopped onion

2 packed cups baby spinach, chard, or kale (or a mix of these)

1 cup fresh peas

Salt and black pepper to taste

Preheat your oven to 400°F. In a bowl, whisk together eggs, milk, and cheeses to combine. Set bowl aside. Place olive oil in an oven-safe skillet (such as cast-iron) and heat over medium heat. Add the onion and sauté until the pieces are clear. Add the greens and peas and turn to coat. Cook until the greens are wilted. Season with salt and pepper, then pour the egg mixture evenly over the greens. Cook until the eggs are partially set. Place the skillet into the oven and bake for 15 minutes.

Serve with a slice of rustic bread for a sustaining meal. Makes 6 servings.

ஐ *Cheesy Kale Pasta*

10–12 leaves of kale or swiss chard, washed and chopped

4 cups whole milk

2 tablespoons olive oil

4 tablespoons butter

1 cup chopped yellow onion

6 tablespoons flour

2 cups shredded monterey jack cheese

8 ounces shell pasta, cooked according to package directions

Salt and pepper to taste

Fill a large pot with water. Add the chopped kale or chard and cook until tender, about 7 minutes. Transfer the greens to a colander and set them aside to drain.

In a small pan, heat milk to scald.

In a skillet, add the olive oil and butter and heat over medium heat. Add the onion and sauté until clear, about 6 minutes. Whisk in the flour and cook for several minutes, stirring constantly. Then add the hot milk and bring to a low boil, whisking continuously. Cook about 6 minutes so the mixture begins to thicken. Remove the skillet from heat and stir in the cheese. Add the kale and cooked pasta and season to taste with salt and pepper. Makes 6 servings.

Protein-Rich Vegetables

As you've probably noticed, I am an advocate for embracing a diet heavy in vegetables. Vegetables are loaded with vitamins. They contain essential minerals and antioxidants necessary for maintaining good health, but the one essential nutrient many lack is protein. Getting enough protein is essential for many processes. In fact, USDA health experts tell us about one quarter of each of our meals should comprise protein-dense foods. You don't have to eat meat to satisfy the demand. There are many meat alternatives rich in protein. Foods like rice, beans, nuts, eggs, dairy, and lentils provide a meatless source of protein. Even potatoes offer eight grams of protein per one-cup serving.

Proteins contain organic compounds called **amino acids** that our bodies use to build their own proteins to grow muscle, regenerate tissue, and generate energy. In fact, there are twenty essential amino acids our bodies need to maintain good health. While our bodies can produce eleven of these amino acids, the other nine must be ingested from the foods we eat. Most vegetable proteins are incomplete proteins, containing some but not all nine amino acids we need. Others, like rice and beans, when served together, become a **complete protein**, or a source of all nine of the essential amino acids the body needs but cannot produce itself. One-half cup of rice and one-half cup of beans provide seven grams of complete protein.

Then there are the superfoods: quinoa, buckwheat, and amaranth. Each is a complete protein containing all nine essential amino acids, just like meat, fish, eggs, and dairy. My family eats a lot of quinoa. I add it to meals to provide protein. A one-cup serving of cooked quinoa contains 8 grams of protein.

Quinoa is easy to make (you prepare it like rice), and its light, nutty flavor blends well with many roasted vegetables and cheese. Mash cooked quinoa into a baked potato and top with cheese and sour cream for a hot, comforting meal chock-full of protein, or mix cooked quinoa with rice and beans and top with queso fresco, avocado, and pico de gallo for a refreshing meal with the power to make you feel good.

≫ Roasted Eggplant and Quinoa

1 medium eggplant, peeled and cut into 1-inch cubes

1 cup quinoa

2 tablespoons olive oil

1 yellow pepper, seeded and cut in thin strips

1 roma tomato, seeded and dice

1 clove garlic, minced

3 tablespoons lemon juice

1 teaspoon oregano

Salt and pepper to taste

1 cup queso fresco (optional)

Preheat your oven to 400°F. Place the eggplant in a steamer with 1 inch of boiling water and cook until tender, about 15 minutes.

While the eggplant is cooking, prepare quinoa according to the package instructions. Then place the olive oil in a skillet and heat over medium low. Add pepper slices and sauté until the peppers begin to brown. Stir in the tomato, garlic, and lemon juice and cook until fragrant, about 5 minutes. Turn off the heat and stir in the oregano and seasonings. When the eggplant is ready, mash it into the pepper mixture.

To assemble, divide the quinoa between 6 plates. Spoon the mixture over quinoa and serve. Top with crumbled queso if desired. Makes 6 servings.

Resources

Elsen, Michael D., and Patrick O. Brown, "Rapid Global Phaseout of Animal Agriculture Has the Potential to Stabilize Greenhouse Gas Levels for 30 Years and Offset 68 Percent of CO_2 Emissions This Century." *PLoS Climate* 1, no. 2 (2022): e0000010. doi: 10.1371/journal.pclm.0000010.

Humane Society International. "Animal Agriculture and Climate Change." Accessed August 22, 2023. https://www.hsi.org/issues/climate-change/.

Marr, Bernard. "The Biggest Future Trends in Agriculture and Food Production." *Forbes*, January 28, 2022. https://www.forbes.com/sites/bernardmarr/2022/01/28/the-biggest-future-trends-in-agriculture-and-food-production/?sh=45731b3d107a.

USDA. "What Is MyPlate?" MyPlate. Accessed August 22, 2023. https://www.myplate.gov/eat-healty/what-is-myplate.

Saffron in This World and Others

⤚ Linda Raedisch ⤛

I can't remember where or when I first came across the story of Elidyr. I almost included it in my book *The Lore of Old Elfland*, but because it fell outside the geographic boundaries I'd set, I left it out. When I went looking for it again, all I could remember was something about fairies, a golden ball, and a saffron-flavored dessert that the fairies were supposed to enjoy.

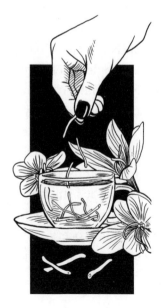

The story of Elidyr, a Welsh boy who stumbled into fairyland and lived to tell the tale, is not a fairy tale or even a folktale—it's a "wonder." Almost a thousand years before podcasters started gathering spooky stories, a handful of monks and clergymen took it upon themsleves to record

accounts of events they couldn't explain. One of these record-
ers was the priest Gerald of Wales, who took down the tale of
another Welsh priest, Elidurus, or Elidyr, as he was known as a
boy. The events in question took place sometime around 1150
in the town of Neath in southern Wales. One day, when his
lessons got too much for the young priest-in-training, young
Elidyr ran away and hid himself in a hollow by the riverbank.

He remained hidden for two days, without food. That's a
long time for a child, so we shouldn't be surprised to hear that
his imagination conjured two small, well-mannered gentlemen to keep up his spirits. The gentlemen were handsome,
wore their hair long, and rode horses the size of greyhounds.
What happened next is indeed surprising. Instead of simply
sitting with him, as hallucinated companions usually do, the
tiny gentlemen took him with them down an underground
passage to their own beautiful country, where he was welcomed by the king and his court as an honored guest.

Elidyr's tiny hosts were, for the most part, vegetarians,
subsisting on junkets and messes of milk and saffron. The fairies people meet in folklore are almost always of a higher so-
cioeconomic class than the mortal, which explains why these
fairies, if fairies they were, were so free with the saffron. To
this day, saffron is the most expensive spice by weight, because
the delicate threads of the saffron crocus—only three per
flower—must be harvested by hand. Don't let this put you off
using it; it's still not as expensive as caviar, and a little goes a
long way. You may find that the saffron in the Hispanic aisle
of your grocery store is much cheaper than the saffron that
comes in little glass jars in the baking aisle.

The saffron "threads" are the stigma of the pale purple saffron crocus, *Crocus sativa*, a fall-blooming flower native to the Middle East. There are only three stigma per flower, which is why they are so precious. By Elidyr's time, saffron was well known in northern Europe, but it was still considered exotic. Both Elidyr and Gerald may have subscribed to the story that the first saffron bulb to reach the British Isles was smuggled out of the Holy Land in the head of a pilgrim's staff, but it's more likely that the Romans introduced it.

Long before the Romans, wild saffron crocuses grew on the Greek island of Santorini. In the 1960s, excavation of a house in the ancient town of Akrotiri revealed a colorful fresco showing young girls with fashionable partially shaven heads gathering purple crocuses on a hillside. The stigma would perhaps have been used as a seasoning, but for the most part, saffron was used to dye cloth and to brew a tea to relieve period cramps. Because of its association with menstruation, saffron-dyed clothing was reserved for women. Because the dye was so precious, it was reserved for royal women and goddesses. In classical times, the goddess Athena, or her idol, wore a saffron-dyed robe that took two priestesses nine months to weave. The fresco of the saffron gatherers survived thanks to a cataclysmic volanic eruption that buried the town in ash around 1600 BCE—the same eruption that gave birth to the legend of Atlantis and its destruction.

I can't resist noting here that Elidyr spent enough time among the saffron-eating fairies of Neath that he started to pick up their language. Upon hearing a sampling of it, including the words for water and salt (but not, unfortunately, for saffron), Gerald of Wales concluded that the fairies' tongue was related to Ancient Greek. Could Elidyr's fairies have been the descendants of Atlantian refugees? Probably not, since there is nothing to suggest that the ancient Santorians were anything less than normal size. Still, it's a fun idea.

Saffron Tea

Today, Spain is the biggest grower of saffron crocuses, and saffron remains a fixture in Hispanic kitchens in America. It hasn't done so well in Anglo kitchens. When I looked up saffron in the index of my trusty copy of *The New Good Housekeeping Cookbook*, I found only two recipes: one for a scallop dish, one for baked rice, and none for "junkets" or "messes." Saffron's popularity picks up again in Iranian kitchens, and if you keep moving east, you'll find it as the beloved key ingredient of a Kashmiri wintertime ritual: *kahwa*, or saffron tea.

Traditionally, kahwa tea is brewed in a *samovar*, a silver, brass, or bronze pot with a "chimney" inside for keeping the tea hot. Yes, *samovar* is a Russian word for a Russian invention, but it's so convenient—hot tea all day long!—that its use has spread far and wide. (The only samovar I've met in person was on a dining-room table belonging to a Russian-American family whose dog I used to walk. Sadly, I never saw it in use.) If you don't have a samovar, you can keep your saffron tea hot in an ordinary teapot with a tea warmer under it. Or you can simply drink it right away. Kahwa enthusiasts say that it is good for digestion, keeps you healthy, helps relieve stress, and makes your skin glow. After all that, I wondered if it could really taste good too, but it does. The honey offsets the bitterness of the green tea and brings out the slight mustiness of the saffron.

✎ *Kahwa*

"A goodly pinch" of saffron threads. Most recipes say to use about 8 saffron threads, but because they're brittle and come tangled together, I use the pinch method. They have a clean, honeyish smell when they're dry, getting mustier as they steep in the hot water.

6 cardamom pods crushed in a mortar and pestle to release the flavor

4 whole cloves

1 cinnamon stick

Water

1 green tea bag or 1 tablespoon loose-leaf green tea. I'm partial to Taiwan high mountain tea, but you can use any green tea as long as it's not flavored.

2 tablespoons honey

Rose petals (optional)

Drop the the saffron threads in a teapot and add just enough boiling water to cover them. Let stand.

Put the cardamom, cloves, and cinnamon stick in a pot with 4½ cups water and bring to a boil. Simmer uncovered for 10 minutes. Add the tea leaves and let sit 2 minutes. Place a sieve over the mouth of the teapot and pour the tea in. Stir in the honey and serve immediately. Garnish each cup with rose petals, dried or fresh, if desired. Serves 4.

Junkets

Now, about those saffron-flavored junkets and messes Elidyr's friends were eating in Faerie: a **mess** is simply a portion or dish of food, while a **junket** is a sweet dish made of milk thickened with rennet. Rennet is made of enzymes drawn from the stomach lining of juvenile ruminants, such as calves, but you can also buy plant-based rennet. Rennet is also used to make cheese. The word *junket* comes to us via Italian or Old French from the Latin *juncus*, a "rush"—any of a number of water-loving plants with long, tapering leaves that, in the old days, were used for making baskets and floor mats, for scouring pots, and as lampwicks. A junket, then, was a thick, creamy food that was poured into a rush basket to set. It must have been a special-occasion dish because it eventually lent its name to any kind of feast and then to an excursion paid for from the public purse.

The saffron crocus, Crocus sativa, *is not to be confused with the autumn crocus, or meadow saffron, which also blooms in autumn, is also purple, and looks a lot like a true crocus. Autumn crocuses actually belong to the genus* Colchicum *and are poisonous.*

Though shorter, crocus leaves are not unlike rush leaves. I once made a very nice bracelet out of ordinary crocus leaves. I braided the leaves while they were green, and they dried to a pretty golden brown. The bracelet lasted for years. In fact, I think I still have it somewhere. Elidyr's fairies could have poured their junkets into little baskets woven from the same saffron crocuses they used to flavor their food.

My own path to junket-making was fraught with peril. Finding a recipe was easy—there are plenty of them online. Finding the rennet tablets was not. Hint: if you ask for "junket rennet tablets" at your grocery store's customer service counter, you'll get farther than if you just ask for "rennet." My favorite store acknowledged that yes, such a product did exist, and that if they had it, it would be with the canning supplies. It wasn't, so I ordered it online. Junket was apparently "a thing" in the 1970s, and my older friends and relatives were familiar with it, though none had made it themselves. My mother, who grew up on raw milk, questioned whether I would be able to make junket with ordinary, grocery store milk. "Of course I will," I told her. "Why wouldn't I?"

I proceeded with my junket. It smelled good when I was cooking it, and the crushed saffron gave it a lovely golden yellow color. It tasted good when I dipped my finger in. I poured it into bowls and waited. It never set, even after two hours in the refrigerator. My mother was right: you can't make junket with ultra-pasteurized milk. Whatever microscopic life forms are supposed to tango with the enzymes in the rennet are not present in treated milk. I include the recipe below for anyone who is lucky enough to have a pipeline to a raw milk supply. Let me know how it goes!

> *Elidyr's Saffron Junket*
>   1 teaspoon rennet or 1 rennet tablet
>   ⅛ cup distilled water
>   2 cups whole milk
>   2 tablespoons sugar
>   "A goodly pinch" saffron threads, crushed in a mortar and
>   pestle

Dissolve the rennet in ⅛ cup distilled water. It will take a while for the tablet to fully dissolve. Stir often to encourage it.

In a double boiler or pot inside another pot filled with water, heat the milk to lukewarm but not quite simmering. Add sugar and saffron and stir until sugar is dissolved. Stir in the dissolved rennet and pour into 4 dessert bowls. Let them sit at room temperature until firm, then chill for 1 hour. Serves 4.

Remember the rose petals I suggested you scatter over your saffron tea? In Kashmir, sliced dried fruit, chopped pistachioes, and slivered almonds are also often sprinkled over *kahwa*. Because I didn't find the idea of chewing and sipping at the same time appealing, I left them out. I suggest you use them here to top your junket. You might add a sprinkle of sugar, cinnamon, and nutmeg too.

Elidyr's Fate

And what, you may ask, happened to Elidyr? He spent many happy days among his new, diminutive friends. For a time, he was able to pass freely between the fairy realm and ours to pay visits to his mother. One day, she asked him for some proof of this strange, subterranean world where he was spending so much of his time. To please her, he brought her a golden ball from the fairy king's court. One can only wonder how things might have gone if Elidyr had asked politely to borrow the ball or had organized a proper "junket" from the palace to his mother's kitchen. Alas, he stole the ball. When the tiny king's men realized what their honored guest had done, they set off in hot pursuit, snatching the ball from Elidyr's hands before he could deliver it to his mother. Then they disappeared. Though he searched for more than a year, Elidyr was never able to find the passage back to Faerie. Even as an old man, whenever he was questioned about his experience, he would weep for shame and for all he had lost.

Resources

Barber, Elizabeth Wayland. *Women's Work: The First 20,000 Years*. New York: W. W. Norton, 1994. Note: oddly, Barber refers to the flowers in the Akrotiri fresco as "saffron lilies."

"Devonshire Junket." *Taste Buds*. Accessed July 30, 2023. https://tastebudsmagazine.co.uk/recipe/devonshire-junket/.

"Frequently Asked Questions." Junket. July 30, 2023. https://junketdesserts.com/faq.

Harris, Elatia. "Saffron Culture: A Pictorial Cycle on Santorini, Part I." *Rambling Epicure* (blog), September 25, 2013. https://www.theramblingepicure.com/tag/saffron-gatherers/.

Mathur, Neha. "Kashmiri Kahwa Tea." *Whisk Affair* (blog), October 3, 2022. https://www.whiskaffair.com/authentic-kashmiri-tea-kahwa-recipe/.

Nazki, Roohi. "Roohi's Zafran Kahwa (Kashmiri Saffron Tea)." Diaspora Co. Accessed July 19, 2023. https://www.diasporaco.com/blogs/recipes/kashmiri-zafran-kahwa-saffron-tea.

Powell, Jessica. "Weird Wales: The Adventure of Elidyr." *Babi a Fi* (blog), March 8, 2023. https://www.babiafi.co.uk/2023/03/weird-wales-adventure-of-elidyr.html.

Spring's Rising: Herbal Vinegars

⇗ Mandana Boushee ⇖

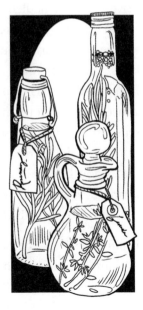

Here in the Northern Hemisphere, the earth is waking from its long winter rest. The skunk cabbages are springing through what's left of the snow, the cottonwood trees are blooming with their Muppet-esque crimson catkins, and the mysterious and striking spring ephemerals are emerging along the forest floor.

If we reflect the state of our health in the seasons, in winter, we adjust to the cold and long nights by eating warm, rich, slow-cooked foods that are often high in fat. This craving for fat is old wiring laced into our DNA from our earliest ancestors, who subsisted on a hunter-gatherer diet. Though we may have easier access to fat sources, shelter, and heat, cold weather still signals to us a need to consume and store extra calories.

Come spring, our bodies shift and adjust to the warmer weather and sunlight. We may find ourselves extra active, sweating more, and beginning to crave less rich foods, maybe even eating significantly less come the hotter months. These spring rhythms and rituals help our bodies balance out from sluggishness, low energy, and poor digestion, which can be side effects of winter.

Spring is also a potent time for plants: as they wake from dormancy, their energy and vital force moves from their underground parts to their aboveground parts. Early spring is an ideal time to harvest tree medicine (buds, bark, resin, flowers) and the underground parts of plants including burdock, yellow dock, dandelion, and Japanese knotweed. Mid to late spring marks the unfurling of the aboveground parts of plants (shoots, leaves, flowers, fiddleheads) that we can harvest too.

In traditional Chinese medicine, spring represents the wood element and is associated with the liver, gallbladder, eyes, tendons, and joints. Many of the plants emerging in the spring are bitter, herbaceous, sour, pungent, mineral rich, and nutrient dense, aiding in supporting our digestion; bone, teeth, nail, and hair health; and the absorption of vitamins and minerals.

Those first spring plants that emerge are, in a sense, the ideal food one needs after a long winter. So it is that most spring herbs encase one or more of these herbal actions, as described by herbalist David Hoffmann:

Lymphatic: These herbs have an ability to move lymph and
    can increase lymphatic flow, moving fluid and protein

away from areas of inflammation so that fresh lymph (rich in oxygen and nutrients needed for tissue repair) can replace it.

Bitter: Bitter herbs help stimulate appetite and digestion by encouraging the production of gastric fluids and peristalsis. The bitter action has a broad action on tone and function, which is effective in activating the production of beneficial digestive secretions, including saliva, gastric acid, and bile.

Alterative: These gradually restore proper functioning of the body and support the metabolic process, increasing health and vitality. Some alteratives support natural waste elimination via the kidneys, liver, lungs, or skin. Others stimulate digestive function or are antimicrobial. These herbs support your body's own natural defenses in the presence of illness and help restore proper function.

Nutritive Tonics: These herbs are high in vitamins and minerals that work to tone the body, providing substance for the building of strength and function of a particular organ or organ system. Tonic herbs correct deficiency and weakness through the vital nourishment of an organ or organ system.

Spring-Centered Herbs

There is an abundance of wonderful plants to harvest for food and medicine come spring. Some of my favorites are bioregional and plentiful where I live in the Northeast, such as nettles, chickweed, cleavers, violets, dandelion greens and roots, spring beauties, clover, burdock root, yellow dock, conifer shoots, and wild onion.

One of the easiest and most delectable ways to harness the high mineral and vitamin content of these plants is to make an herbal vinegar. Vinegar is a fantastic menstruum for extracting minerals and vitamins from plants, as alcohol cannot draw out these constituents. However, you can still make alcohol tinctures with the before-mentioned plants to extract other beneficial and medicinal chemical constituents.

Herbal vinegars are a great alternative to alcohol-based medicines for folks who avoid or refrain from alcohol and for children, and they are generally incredibly affordable to make, especially if you are able to harvest some or all of the plants from your garden, outdoor surroundings, the wild, and so on.

Herbal vinegars differ from oxymels and shrubs in that no honey or sweetener is added to the vinegar. With this in mind, you'll notice in the recipe on pages 109–11 that there are no sweeteners added, but feel free to add honey, maple syrup, or a handful of fruit of your choice if you'd like to sweeten up your batch.

This herbal vinegar recipe centers on local and abundant plants growing in the Northeast, while also incorporating some warming common culinary plants. I've added warming and stimulating plants (ginger, garlic, conifers) to the recipe, as I enjoy a little kick of heat in my vinegars, but feel free to experiment with spices and herbs that feel resonant with your palate.

Herbal Properties of Plants Used in Our Herbal Vinegar

Nettles (*Urtica* spp.)

Actions and Benefits: Nutritive tonic (affinity to kidney and adrenals), astringent, adaptogen, hemostatic, diuretic, natural antihistamine

Parts to Use: Young leaves, seeds, roots

Ways to Incorporate: Tea, tincture, vinegar, syrup, salve, infused oil, as food

Used For: Allergies; urinary tract infections; building blood; promoting lactation; arthritis; asthma; strengthening nails, hair, teeth, bones

Dandelion (*Taraxacum officinale*)

Actions and Benefits: Alterative, nutritive tonic, diuretic, bitter, digestive stimulant, cholagogue

Parts to Use: Roots, leaves, flowers, sap

Ways to Incorporate: Tincture, tea, infused oil, salve, vinegar, food, wine, flower essence

Used For: Liver support and function, gallbladder support and function, eczema, poor digestion, acne, menstrual symptoms, fluid retention, nutrition

Violet (*Viola* spp.)

Actions and Benefits: Lymphatic, alterative, demulcent, anti-inflammatory, mild pain relief, high in vitamin C

Parts to Use: Leaves and flowers

Ways to Incorporate: Tea, herbal pesto, food, tincture, infused oil, vinegar, syrup, cordial, flower essence

Used For: Chest health; swollen lymph glands; lymph support; sore throats; pain relief; teething; eczema; hot, irritated rashes; sunburn; arthritis; emotional heart support; eye wash

Burdock (*Arctium* spp.)

Actions and Benefits: Alterative, diuretic, nutritive tonic, lymphatic, hepatic, high in inulin

Parts to Use: Root, seed, leaf

Ways to Incorporate: Tea, tincture, poultice, as food, vinegar, infused oil, lactofermented root

Used For: A wide range of skin ailments (dry, scaly skin; oily skin; acne; eczema; rashes), allergies, mold allergies, supporting liver health, aiding digestive health, fluid retention, nutrition, urinary system support, lymphatic support, elimination function support

Yellow Dock (*Rumex* spp.)

Actions and Benefits: Alterative, high in iron, bitter, astringent

Parts to Use: Root, leaves (in small amounts, as the leaves are high in oxalic acid)

Ways to Incorporate: Tea, food, tincture, syrup, vinegar

Used For: Anemia, constipation, diarrhea, healthy digestion, cooling liver heat, skin ailments

Cleavers (*Galium aparine*)

Actions and Benefits: Lymphatic, alterative, vulnerary, diuretic, anti-inflammatory

Parts to Use: Leaves

Ways to Incorporate: Tea, soup, tincture, vinegar, salve, poultice, food

Used For: Skin ailments, sunburn, burns, lymphatic support, urinary tract infections

Pine (*Pinus* spp.)

Actions and Benefits: Astringent, warming, aromatic, high in vitamin C, expectorant

Parts to Use: Needles, pitch, cones, pollen

Ways to Incorporate: Tea, syrup, salve, oil, chest rubs, flower essence, tincture

Used For: Cold and flu, productive coughs, respiratory infections

Ginger (*Zingiber officinale*)

Actions and Benefits: Stimulating, warming, diffusive, expectorant, diaphoretic, improves circulation

Parts to Use: Rhizome

Ways to Incorporate: Decoction, ginger chest rub, warming syrup, warming blends, glycerite, tincture, vinegar, oxymel

Used For: Sore throats, congested coughs, stuffy sinuses, poor circulation, fever, nausea

Garlic (*Allium sativum*)

Actions and Benefits: Antibiotic, antiviral, antiseptic, warming, stimulating

Parts to Use: Bulb

Ways to Incorporate: Soup, food, infused oil, infused honey, vinegar mouth rinse, fire cider, poultice

Used For: Common cold, bronchitis, flu, respiratory infections, circulation, earache, blood pressure

Spring Herbal Vinegar Recipe

Typically, dried herbs are much more potent than fresh material, as dried herbs have zero water content. That is why this recipe calls for less dry material than fresh.

You will need:

> Generous handful of fresh dandelion leaf or 2 tablespoons dried dandelion leaf and roots
>
> Generous handful of fresh burdock roots or 2 tablespoons dried burdock roots (Asian groceries and health food stores often sell fresh burdock root.)
>
> Generous handful of fresh yellow dock roots or 2 tablespoons dried yellow dock roots

Generous handful of fresh nettle leaf or 2 tablespoons dried nettle leaf

Generous handful of fresh violet leaf and flower or 2 tablespoons dried violet leaf and flower

Generous handful of fresh cleavers or 2 tablespoons dried cleavers

Generous handful of fresh or dried conifer medicine, like pine or spruce needles, or 2 tablespoons dried conifer medicine

Ginger (amount desired depends on your preference; the more you add the spicer it will be)

Garlic (amount desired depends on your preference; the more you add the spicer it will be)

Vinegar of choice and availability

Jar with a lid

1. Wash your fresh ingredients and pat dry, removing all excess water.
2. Cut your fresh ingredients (dandelion, burdock, yellow dock, nettle, violet, cleavers, conifer, ginger, and garlic) finely. You may also use a food processor. It's important that your herbs are chopped finely to increase the surface area of the plant.
3. Place your cut ingredients (fresh and dried) into the jar and cover with vinegar, making sure that all your plant material is fully submerged in the vinegar.
4. Place the jar in a cool, dark place, checking on it daily to make sure the plant material is still immersed in the vinegar, topping off with vinegar if needed.
5. After a few weeks, strain the vinegar and use it as you desire.

After a couple of days, you may notice a white cloudy substance at the bottom of your jar. This is completely okay! Dandelion and burdock are both high in **inulin**. Inulin is a starch-like substance that isn't digestible by humans but provides food for the bacteria in our gut. You will often hear people refer to inulin as a prebiotic for this reason. It's also important to note that if you ingest large amounts of inulin, you may have gas and bloating. If you are a person who has sensitivities or allergies to foods like Jerusalem artichokes, asparagus, garlic, or onions (all foods high in inulin), please consider using less or omitting dandelion, burdock, and garlic from your herbal vinegar.

How to Use Your Herbal Vinegar

There is a multitude of ways to use and incorporate your spring herbal vinegar into your routine. You can weave your finished vinegar into food applications, such as these:

- Salad dressings
- Steaming your greens or vegetables with a dash of the vinegar, or adding it to cooked greens or vegetables
- Adding the vinegar to rich soups and broths for a bit of acidity
- Adding the vinegar and a bit of a sweetener to soda water for a refreshing shrub

You can incorporate your spring vinegar in more medicinal applications:

- Taking a tablespoon before and after meals to aid in digestion

- Taking a tablespoon throughout the day on the onset of a cold
- Taking when you feel sluggish, nauseous, or low energy
- Using the vinegar topically for weepy rashes like poison ivy, poison sumac, and eczema

You can also incorporate your spring vinegar in beauty applications:

- Soaking a cotton ball in the vinegar and applying to your face as a toner
- Using the vinegar as a hair wash for itchy scalp

Resource

Hoffmann, David. *The Herbal Handbook: A User's Guide to Medical Herbalism*. Rochester, VT: Healing Arts Press, 1988.

Preserving Fruits and Flowers

❧ Marilyn I. Bellemore ❧

I've always been attuned to the seasons and calendar year. It was something that came naturally to me as a child growing up in southern New England. When the first violets popped up in my backyard, I knew it was late February. This meant that snow would be coming to an end, and I should soon expect to see the bright yellow daffodils of March.

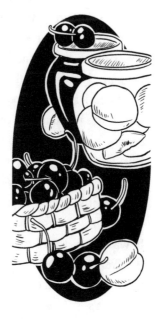

The excitement for me was not only the beauty of it all, but that I could eat many of the fruits and flowers that grew wild in my yard. The leaves of the clover plant were a favorite with their sweet, grassy taste, devoured fresh and unwashed. Strawberries grew on the same small hill on the side of my house. My mom made sure to grab enough handfuls for several pies to complement the rhubarb our neighbor Mr. Miller gave us each June. But the most fun for me was pinching the base of the flower off a honeysuckle tree that provided a sweet drop of pure delight.

I am now lucky to live part of the time on a farm in the Green Mountains of Vermont that offers the magic of my childhood in the fruits and flowers that grow here. Each spring, I look out the window and see blankets of deep yellow dandelions followed by a sea of buttercups in a lighter hue. Every couple of weeks through the fall, there's a different wildflower flower growing or tree blossoming in the fields. I am careful to note what can and can't be eaten, as well as the right time to harvest the crop for my jellies, jams, syrups, and butters.

Nothing is more satisfying than spearmint jelly served alongside roast lamb in the autumn, blueberry lime jam on my morning crostini in the winter, pear butter grilled cheese for a springtime lunch, or fresh-squeezed lemonade sweetened with lilac syrup in the summer. I always share the abundance with family and friends, and it seems everyone has a favorite that they look forward to each year.

Wild fruit trees grow randomly on my property, which inspired me to plant my own small orchard, including additional cherry, peach, pear, apple, and plum trees. I'm from Smithfield, Rhode Island, which is the apple capital of the state. Early on, I became a big fan of 'Macoun' and 'Granny Smith' and thought I knew just about every apple that existed. That was until I bought my house on Prince Edward Island, Canada, in 2019. It was there that I discovered an apple tree in my yard called the 'Yellow Transparent' (or August apple). This versatile apple has been enjoyed on Prince Edward Island since the 1840s. Currently, it's my favorite variety to cook with.

While researching the wild fruit trees that grow on my farm, I discovered a nonprofit organization called the Lost Apple Project. Although its focus is on the Pacific Northwest, I'm intrigued to follow along on its Facebook page and learn about recent findings. The goal is to seek out forgotten apple varieties that once grew on old homesteads and abandoned orchards. Once identified, volunteers take cuttings to graft onto new trees to create a new supply of the lost fruit. I keep my own notebook now and do a thorough walkthrough of my property once a year. Twice in three years, I've found apple trees I didn't know existed and, this year, more blackberry bushes.

Did you know apples, peaches, raspberries, and blackberries are all high in pectin or behave like they are? Because of this, I keep preserving simple and only use these fruits in pectin-free jams or slow-cooker butters.

In Vermont, my September ritual is to go down to the area behind my pond where tiny grapes grow. They're not the cold-hardy type that you'd expect to see. I call them a champagne grape because of their size. One year, I painstakingly juiced them by hand to make jelly. It was delicious yet time consuming. Since I discovered the old-fashioned and less popular way to make grape jam with the skins still on, I've settled on that because it tastes just as nice.

During raspberry season, I pick each day. It's not the traditional pick-your-own method like at the local farm stand. Instead, knee-deep in underbrush, I rummage through thickets in all areas of my yard. By the entrance to the forest and along the old red barn is where they grow best. On days that the local black bear family has been spotted wandering on my remote road, I'll drive the ATV just in case.

And it's not just black bears that enjoy their berries. Today, when I went out to pick blueberries, a bush that was filled ripe and juicy yesterday was surprisingly sparse. It wasn't until I went to check on my seven four-month-old lambs a couple of hours later that I realized they had stuck their tiny mouths through the fence by the bush.

Jam, Syrup, and Butter Recipes

I've perfected my recipes through trial and error. A failed honeysuckle jelly became a now-favorite syrup with which to baste baked ham. On a day when I didn't have time to buy pectin, I created a jam recipe that excluded it.

My methods for canning jellies, jams, syrups, and butters are as follows. I use what I call "gathering baskets" to harvest as much of the fruits and flowers as possible the second they're ready for picking. Waiting several days can mean all the difference, especially with unpredictable weather in the mountain climate where I live. Often short on time, I learned the hard way never to double a recipe because it simply won't work. Surface area for evaporation is reduced, the resulting increased cook time can ruin texture or setting, and most home cooks lack equipment for larger-scale canning, making doubling inadvisable and at the very least unreliable.

Depending on what I'm making, the fruits and flowers are "picked through" to remove any debris, then rinsed in cold water. Next, either I make them into a tea and steep overnight, or I ready the fruit if it needs peeling and chopping, like apples and pears. Then I begin the canning process. My suggestion is to take your time when following recipes, and eventually, with patience, you'll be able to shorten the time it takes you by half.

Even if you don't live on a farm or grow your own edible fruits and flowers, jam ingredients are often within close reach. I find supermarkets price fruits on sale when they are about to "turn." This is a great way to buy often-overpriced cherries and berries to make jams. Next time you're out for an afternoon walk or drive, notice fields of dandelions or the smell of spearmint along creeks and rivers in season. Do lilac bushes or honeysuckle trees grow in or around your neighborhood? If they do and are on private property, asking the owner permission to pick a few cups of flowers in exchange for a jar of flavorful jelly might be an excellent barter.

Once you begin canning, feel free to experiment with flavors by mixing and matching. For example, if I have lemon balm on hand, I might add it along with a recipe that requires spearmint. I sometimes substitute lemon juice with lime juice when using blueberries to kick the flavor up a notch. What follows are simple instructions for some of my favorite jellies, jams, syrups, and butters. These basic recipes can be used as templates for preserving a variety of fruits and flowers—try them out and customize them throughout your preserve-making journey to make them your own.

☙ Basic Jelly Recipe (with Pectin)

This recipe works great for flowers and herbs such as dandelion, lilac, honeysuckle, and spearmint. I like to make and steep the tea for these jellies as soon as I pick the flowers or leaves.

You will need:

- 2 cups dandelion petals (remove the green part of the flower), lilac flowers, honeysuckle flowers, or spearmint leaves, lightly packed
- 4 cups water
- 4 cups sugar
- 2 tablespoons lemon juice
- 1 box powdered pectin

Place the petals into a quart canning jar or metal pitcher.

Pour 4 cups of boiling water over the flower petals. Allow the liquid to cool and then place it in the fridge for 24 hours.

Strain the flowers well and squeeze out as much tea as possible.

Place 3½–4 cups of tea, the lemon juice, and pectin into a large pot. Bring it to a boil.

Add sugar and return to a boil while stirring. Boil the jelly for 1 to 2 minutes.

Remove from heat and pour or ladle the jelly into sterilized canning jars. Process for 10 minutes in a boiling water bath canner or simply boil the jars in the pan of water you sterilized them in for 10 minutes. Makes about 4 half-pint jars or 8 quarter-pint jars that should keep for about 2 years.

⁂ Basic Jam Recipe (No Pectin)

Try this recipe for strawberry, blueberry, raspberry, blackberry, grape, cherry, or plum jam. If I don't have enough of one type of berry for a batch on a given day, I will mix different ones together for what I call "fruits of the farm."

You will need:

- 4 cups berries, grapes (seeds removed), cherries (pitted and chopped), or plums (pitted and chopped)
- 3 cups sugar
- 2 tablespoons lemon juice

Mash the fruit until desired consistency.

Put all ingredients into a medium saucepan and stir to combine. Place on medium heat until mixture comes to a boil. Reduce heat and boil about 15–20 minutes.

Follow canning procedure in the basic jelly recipe. Makes about 4 half-pint jars or 8 quarter-pint jars that should keep for about 2 years.

℘ Basic Syrup Recipe

Make an herbal or floral syrup with this customizable basic recipe. These syrups are delightful to sweeten teas or lemonades. I like to use dandelion, lilac, honeysuckle, or spearmint.

You will need:

- 2 cups sugar
- 1 cup water
- 1 cup flower petals (remove the green part of the dandelion flower) or spearmint leaves

Dissolve the sugar in water in a saucepan over medium heat, stirring occasionally, until it reaches a simmer. Put the flowers or leaves in a heat-resistant bowl. Pour the hot syrup over the top and let stand for at least 30 minutes. Strain the mixture and discard flowers or leaves. Makes roughly 2¼ cups.

Some people pour the syrup into clean stopper bottles. It will keep in the fridge for about 1 month, or you can can it. I follow the same canning process as with jellies and jams but use wide-mouth mason jars.

⚛ Basic Slow Cooker Butter Recipe
This actually isn't butter at all. The origin of the name is simply the consistency, and this "butter" is delicious on breads, as a side dish with meats, or in recipes that call for applesauce. Try this recipe with apples, pears, peaches, or plums.

You will need:
- 3 cups peeled, cored, and chopped apples, pears, peaches, or plums of your choice
- ½ cup sugar
- ½ cup light brown sugar
- 1 teaspoon ground cinnamon
- ¼ teaspoon allspice
- ¼ teaspoon nutmeg

Place the fruit in a slow cooker. Top with sugar, brown sugar, cinnamon, allspice, and nutmeg and mix well.

Cover and cook on high for 4–5 hours and stir occasionally until the fruit is dark brown and tender.

Spoon the finished butter into containers or jars, cover, and refrigerate. Makes about 4 half-pint jars or 8 quarter-pint jars.

Cooling Herbs

Elizabeth Barrette

In high temperatures, the body often struggles to keep up with demands. Sweating can lower body temperature, but it costs water. Enter cooling herbs. They use a variety of methods to help people cool off. Some, like celery, contain lots of water. Some, such as hibiscus, offer electrolytes without sodium. Others, like spearmint, actually smell, taste, and feel cold—sometimes called "minty," "medicinal," or "camphoraceous" scents. All of these make them helpful for comfort and health in hot weather.

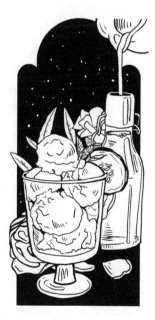

Herbs with Cooling Effects

Numerous herbs are known for cooling effects. They appear often in spring and summer dishes. Many are used to flavor beverages as well. Some are easy to grow at home, while others are a bit more challenging or just better to buy. Take a look at some of the most popular cooling herbs.

Amchur

Amchur (*Mangifera indica*) is a sweet-tart powder made from dried green mango fruit. You may find dried amchur slices too. As mango trees grow quite large and require a tropical environment, most people buy amchur at an international food store. It has antibacterial, antioxidant, anti-inflammatory, and other medicinal qualities. It's used as a souring agent in Indian and other Southeast Asian cuisines.

Celery

Celery (*Apium graveolens*) can be grown as a vegetable (with thick stems and few leaves) or an herb (with thin stems and many leaves) depending on the cultivar. You may grow it at home, but people often prefer to buy it for convenience. Rich in vitamins and mineral salts, it also holds a lot of water and is good to consume after sweating. It has antimicrobial, antioxidant, anti-inflammatory, and other medicinal qualities. Celery appears in hot and cold soups, cold snacks, and beverages.

Cilantro

Cilantro (*Coriandrum sativum*) is a leafy green herb. *Cilantro* refers to the leaves and *coriander* to the seeds, and different cultivars emphasize each of those. It is easy to grow, even in a windowbox. Some people find that cilantro tastes like soap, so they may substitute relatives such as parsley. It's widely used as a salad green and for condiments such as pesto, salsa, and dips. Cilantro has analgesic, antimicrobial, antioxidant, anti-inflammatory, and digestive properties.

Cucumber

Cucumber (*Cucumis sativus*) is thought of more as a vegetable than an herb, but its strong cooling qualities allow it to function as an herbal agent. It combines well with other herbs in salads or beverages for cold meals in hot weather. Easy to grow, it's one of the most common garden plants. High in electrolytes and vitamins, cucumber also has antioxidant, anti-inflammatory, and other medicinal qualities.

Dill

Dill (*Anethum graveolens*) is a tall, feathery herb with finely divided leaves. Both the leaves and the seeds can be used. It has a bright, tangy flavor that goes well with fish or chicken. Easy to grow, it's common in herb gardens, and the leaves are better fresh. Dill has antimicrobial, soothing, and digestive qualities.

Fennel

Fennel (*Foeniculum vulgare*) has several subspecies, including sweet fennel, bronze fennel, bulb fennel, and wild pepper fennel. It tends to have a licorice flavor, and can be grown for its feathery leaves or thick bulb. It is relatively easy to grow. Fennel has digestive, antimicrobial, antinausea, and energizing properties.

Hibiscus

Hibiscus is a beautiful red flower whose sepals can be dried for use in tea, tinctures, or jams. The petals are edible too. African and diaspora users favor *Hibiscus sabdariffa*, while traditional Chinese medicine prefers *H. rosa-sinensis*. Hibiscus is moderately easy to grow in the right climate and looks spectacular in the garden. It provides electrolytes along with antibacterial, antioxidant, and soothing qualities.

Lavender

Lavender is a gray-green herb with blue to purple flowers. Among the more popular types are English lavender (*Lavandula angustifolia*), French lavender (*L. dentata*), Spanish lavender (*L. stoechas*), and various hybrids. Widely prized for scenting soap, perfume, and other toiletries, lavender flowers are edible and may be used to make purple syrups and sorbets or for French cuisine. Some people think it tastes like soap, though. It's easier to grow your own, and that way you know it's safe—otherwise, make sure you buy culinary lavender, not craft supplies. It has analgesic, antimicrobial, calming, cleansing, digestive, and soporific qualities.

Lemongrass

Lemongrass (*Cymbopogon citratus*) has narrow blade-like leaves with a fleshy base and a strong citrusy smell. Dried leaves may be used in teas or soups, but the fleshy base is often chopped into stir-fries or minced as an aromatic. It is not difficult to grow, but it requires a tropical climate, so temperate gardeners may grow it in a container that can be overwintered indoors. Lemongrass has antimicrobial, digestive, nervine, and other medicinal properties.

Mint

Mint is a low bushy herb that comes in many forms. Popular types include apple mint (*Mentha suaveolens*), chocolate mint (*M. ×piperita* f. *citrata* 'Chocolate'), garden mint (*M. canadensis*), spearmint (*M. spicata*), and peppermint (*M. ×piperita*). Many are notorious for spreading, so grow each type of mint in its own container or a bed with solid walls. Mint goes in everything from salads to ice cream to beverages and is especially valuable for cutting the heaviness of rich foods like lamb. It has antibacterial, antinausea, antioxidant, digestive, invigorating, and other medicinal qualities.

Parsley

Parsley is a small leafy green herb that has several main types. These include curly parsley (*Petroselinum crispum* var. *crispum*), flat-leaf parsley (*P. crispum* var. *neapolitanum*), Japanese parsley (*Cryptotaenia japonica*), and root parsley (*P. crispum*). Most are grown for the leaves, except for root parsley. Easy to grow, flat and curly are the most common in gardens. Its dark green leaves are packed with vitamins. Parsley has antimicrobial, anti-inflammatory, and digestive properties.

Rose

Rose is a small to medium bush whose flower petals and hips may be used. There are over a hundred species and countless hybrids. For culinary and medicinal uses, many prefer the fragrant old-garden varieties or else wild roses. Good choices include apothecary rose (*Rosa gallica*), cabbage rose (*R. ×centifolia*), damask rose (*R. ×damascena*), dog rose (*R. canina*), rugosa rose *(R. rugosa)*, and white rose (*R. ×alba*). These are also easier to grow than fussy modern hybrids—easiest of all if you select a wild rose native to your locale. Rose petals may be candied, dried for use in tea, or made into roseflower water. The hips are most often turned into syrup or jelly, but they can be used in tea and have abundant vitamin C. Rose has antibacterial, antioxidant, relaxing, and other medicinal qualities.

Refreshing Recipes with Cooling Herbs

Herbs with cooling qualities make food refreshing, ideal for hot weather. They combine well with many juicy things. Because they lean toward cleansing or antimicrobial properties, they also help discourage pests and spoilage, which makes them a much better choice for picnics than egg-based or dairy-based dishes that spoil quickly in the heat. They also stay cool and refreshing longer once you take them out of the refrigerator. Electrolytes in some of these herbs replenish those lost to sweat. If you use salt, favor sea salt or mineral salt to maximize trace elements, but if you want to minimize salt, just look for the cooling herbs high in nonsodium electrolytes, such as potassium, and use those instead. Note that leafy green herbs of cooling character tend to substitute well. If you dislike cilantro, you can swap in parsley or celery leaves for most recipes.

⤝ Fantastic Flower Salad

   1 cup fresh rose petals, hibiscus sepals, and/or lavender
      petals (or other edible flowers)
   ½ cup fresh leaves of cilantro, dill, fennel, mint, and/or
      parsley (or other herbs)
   2–3 cups lettuce, baby spinach leaves, and/or spring mix
      salad greens
   ½ cup sliced cucumber
   ¼ cup diced celery

Toss together the flower petals, herb leaves, and lettuce or other salad greens. Put a handful of the salad mix in a large bowl, sprinkle on some cucumber and celery, then repeat the layering process with the rest of the ingredients. This prevents the chunks from drifting to the bottom. You may add other salad ingredients, such as tomatoes or sunflower seeds, if you wish. When you can find fresh lemongrass shoots, shave them thin and add them along with the cucumber.

If you want dressing, choose a light fruity one such as raspberry vinaigrette to avoid drowning out the colors and flavors of the flowers and herbs. If you like your salad with just a sprinkle of flavored vinegar and good olive oil, or a "naked salad" dusted with a spice blend, this is perfect for those too. Makes about 4 servings.

⪢ Refreshing Summer Salad

1½ cups diced cucumber (about 1 cucumber)

½ cup diced heirloom tomato (about 1 beefsteak or 6 cherry tomatoes)

¼ cup chopped cilantro, celery, mint, and/or flat-leaf parsley leaves

Toss everything together, chill, and serve. For a sweeter salad, you may replace some or all of the cucumber with another green or white melon such as honeydew. Makes about 4 servings.

⪢ Cooling Pesto

1 cup celery, cilantro, mint, and/or flat-leaf parsley leaves

1 tablespoon nuts and/or seeds (pine nuts, walnuts, sunflower seeds, etc.)

1 teaspoon lime or lemon juice

1 garlic clove (or ½ teaspoon garlic paste)

1 tablespoon hard grating cheese (parmesan, pecorino, manchego, etc.)

4 tablespoons oil (olive, walnut, sunflower, etc.)

Pinch of sea salt or bamboo salt

Combine all ingredients. Mash to a paste with a mortar and pestle, or use an appliance such as a blender or food processor to puree everything. Makes 3–4 servings as a pasta topping or more as a condiment.

This basic pesto recipe easily adapts to whatever ingredients you have. You can also substitute flavored vinegar for the citrus juice. If you dislike garlic, try using minced lemongrass shoots as the aromatic. Spread the pesto on sandwiches, toss with pasta or vegetables, use as salad dressing, or pour over grilled meat such as chicken or fish.

ꙮ Tangy Masala Potatoes

   1 tablespoon amchur powder

   1 tablespoon turmeric

   2 teaspoons ground cumin

   2 teaspoons ground coriander

   ½ teaspoon sea salt or pink salt

   1 pound potatoes

   ¼ cup chopped cilantro or parsley leaves

   1 lime or lemon, quartered

To make the masala, simply mix together all the powdered spices. If you want to get fancy, you can use whole cumin and coriander seeds, toasting them before grinding them. Store the blend in a glass spice jar.

The potatoes can be made in various ways. For a non-dairy, picnic-friendly potato salad, simply boil potatoes and cube them, mix 1 tablespoon of masala with enough tahini to make a sauce, and toss everything together. If you're grilling, thread potato chunks on skewers, brush with oil, dust with masala, and grill until tender. If you have an air fryer, slice or chunk the potatoes, toss with masala and a little oil, then follow your appliance's directions for air-frying vegetables. Once done, you can dress up the potatoes with chopped cilantro or parsley leaves and a squeeze of lemon or lime juice. Makes 2–3 servings.

This masala also works well for seasoning other mild vegetables like sunchokes or cauliflower, rice, or light meats such as fish or chicken.

ﾞﾞ Cucumber Mint Sorbet

This version is just barely sweet and makes a great palate cleanser or frozen salad. For something more dessert-like, you can increase the sweetener.

You will need:

> 3 cups cucumber chunks (about 2 cucumbers)
>
> 2 tablespoons fresh mint leaves
>
> ⅛ cup organic sugar syrup, agave syrup, or honey
>
> Pinch of sea salt or bamboo salt
>
> Zest of one lime
>
> ½ teaspoon lime juice

There are various ways to freeze this:

1. If you have an ice cream maker, puree the ingredients together, then pour the mix in the churn and follow your appliance's directions for making sorbet.
2. If you have a high-power blender, you can freeze chunks of cucumber, then put ½ cup water in the bottom of the blender, add the other ingredients, and process until smooth.

3. You can also freeze puree in an ice cube tray, then process that instead of just cucumber chunks. Those ice cubes also work great in agua fresca.
4. If you have a snow-cone maker that can handle flavored ice, you can freeze blocks of puree for it.

Makes about 6 servings.

⁂ Fancy Flower Syrup

Red hibiscus and red to pink rose petals should give you a pink-to-purple syrup; if you use dark purple lavender, it may lean a bit more toward the bluish side of purple.

You will need:

    1 cup water

    1 cup organic sugar

    ½ cup fresh hibiscus sepals

    ½ cup fresh rose petals

    2 tablespoons lavender buds

In a small pot, place the water and sugar, stirring to dissolve. Add the flowers. Heat until it simmers, then cook gently for 5 minutes. Let the syrup cool, then strain into a glass jar. Use this flower syrup to flavor snow cones, make homemade sodas or mixed drinks, pour over ice cream, or dress a fruit salad. Makes about 24 servings.

You can make this with dried petals, but you only need about half as much. For richer color, you may add a tiny amount of red or purple gel food coloring. Another option is more edible flower petals: black (dark purple) pansies usually give a good blue-violet to violet, and you can buy pea flowers for a bright sky blue. You could also make syrup with 1 individual flower flavor, using a whole cup of rose or hibiscus, or 3 tablespoons of lavender.

⪼ Red Drink

The original "red drink" was not a fruity soda, but a hibiscus tea or mixed drink like this, spanning numerous African and diaspora cultures, with countless variations.

You will need:

    2 quarts water
    1 cup dried hibiscus sepals
    1 cup dried rose petals
    1 tablespoon dried lemongrass
    1 cup organic sugar

In a pot, boil the water. Stir in the dried flowers and lemongrass. Remove from the heat and allow to cool completely. Strain the liquid into a pitcher. Add the sugar and stir until dissolved. Taste and adjust sweetness if necessary. Chill and serve over ice. Makes about 8 servings.

Herbal Ice Cubes

    Water
    Edible flower petals
    Herb leaves
    Cucumber slices

For this, you need a tray or mold that makes large ice cubes; you can even find huge square or spherical ones at a well-stocked liquor store or cooking supply store. Fresh rose petals, hibiscus sepals, or whole lavender flower heads work well. For herb leaves, try mint, parsley, or cilantro. Cucumber slices also look good. Fill the tray, tuck a petal or leaf into each hole, and freeze. These make delightful accents to cooling beverages.

Conclusion

Cooling herbs bring relief in hot weather, helping people stay comfortable and maintain the water balance in their bodies. They also help with warm, dry body conditions such as hot flashes or fever. They look beautiful and taste delicious. You can grow many of them in an herb garden—look for a mostly sunny spot that gets a bit of shade from the midday heat. Most dry well enough to store well too. Give them a try!

Health
and
Beauty

Micronutrients in Plant-Based Foods

❧ Mireille Blacke, RD, CD-N ❧

Maintaining a "balanced diet" isn't always easy when following a plant-based lifestyle. To prevent nutritional deficiencies, it becomes extremely important to consider the nutrition content and bioavailability (extent to which nutrients are absorbed by the body) in plant-based food sources, as well as the best ways to prepare and cook them. While most people are familiar with the macronutrient (carbohydrate, fat, and protein) composition of their meal planning, those who eat only plant-based foods would benefit from a solid understanding of the micronutrient (vitamin, mineral, and trace mineral) content of their chosen plant sources.

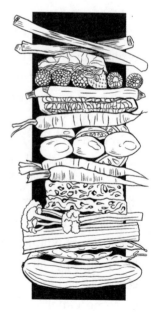

I'll be the first person to say it: talking about food can trigger some obsessive tendencies in people. A registered dietitian, the breed to which I belong, is typically a detail-oriented and evidence-based sort of creature, driven by the latest studies and need to keep well-informed of all things food. However, I've had very "motivated" clients send me meticulously crafted spreadsheets of their own data, including amazingly documented analyses of their own daily micronutrient intake that have made my own research-loving head spin.

While this can be a very complicated topic, let's aim for simplicity and sanity. In this article, I will explain what those plant-based vitamins, minerals, and trace minerals do for the body, offer the best plant-based food sources of specific micronutrients, and discuss how cooking impacts their micronutrient content (e.g., cooked versus raw status). My overall goal with this article is to inform you on the best ways to slow down micronutrient loss from your plant-based food sources, resulting in greater bioavailability and better health.

To further assist with the goal of simplicity, this article won't address the organic versus traditionally grown or locally grown versus chain grocery store arguments, and will not include certain micronutrients for which most Americans easily meet optimal nutritional needs in their daily dietary intakes (e.g., minerals like potassium and sodium). I will not address food intolerance, sensitivity, allergies, or most dietary limitations. With one exception, the topic of micronutrient supplements will not be covered in this article. The topics in this paragraph, along with micronutrient needs during pregnancy and lactation, and particularly individual needs pertaining to potential food and medication interactions should be reviewed by readers with their healthcare provider(s).

The easiest way to tackle micronutrients is as follows: vitamins, minerals, and trace minerals. Vitamins are then categorized as water-soluble and fat-soluble.

I'll use the following format to explain each micronutrient:

Micronutrient Name (Best Known)
Also Known As (AKA)/Best Absorbed Form
Functions in the Body
Plant-Based Sources: Found at significant levels in this micronutrient
Potential Deficiencies: Signs and symptoms, ranging from mild to severe

Water-Soluble Vitamins

If you read an ingredient label on any vitamin or mineral supplement, it's easy to get overwhelmed by the list of tough-to-pronounce compounds that are printed there. The cool part about water-soluble vitamins is that they are made of just B vitamins and vitamin C. That's it! While there are plenty of separate B vitamins, remembering this is less confusing when organizing your micronutrients.

The most important points you need to know about water-soluble vitamins are that they dissolve in water and are not stored for any significant amount of time in the body, which means they must be consumed regularly. This also means that any excess B or C vitamins will be flushed out of the body if unused. When it comes to cooking, water-soluble vitamins also lose the most micronutrients when exposed to heat and most forms of cooking.

Vitamin B$_1$

AKA: Thiamine mononitrate

Functions in the Body: Normal functioning of nervous system, brain, gastrointestinal tract, immune system; carbohydrate to energy metabolism; healthy mood and sleep cycles

Potential Deficiencies: Blurry vision, delirium, fatigue, heart issues, irritability, loss of appetite, paralysis, sleep disturbances

Plant-Based Sources: Acorn squash, beet greens, black beans, brussels sprouts, cardamom, corn, enriched grains and breads, lentils, peas, sunflower seeds

Vitamin B$_2$

AKA: Riboflavin

Functions in the Body: Digestion, energy metabolism, growth, nerve function

Potential Deficiencies: Blurred vision, depression, fatigue, hair loss, light sensitivity, reproductive issues, skin cracking, swollen throat

Plant-Based Sources: Cardamom, whole grains, green vegetables

Vitamin B$_3$

AKA: Niacin, niacinamide

Functions in the Body: Aids nervous system, digestion, skin health, cognitive function, and mood

Potential Deficiencies: Pellagra (dark, scaly rash with bright redness of the tongue), constipation or diarrhea, depression, headache, dementia

Plant-Based Sources: Asparagus, avocado, brown rice, green peas, mushrooms, peanuts, sunflower seeds

Vitamin B_6

AKA: Pyroxidine hydrochloride

Functions in the Body: Aids in muscle contraction and heart
function, blood pressure regulation, cognitive function,
manufacture of body proteins and hormones, normal
serotonin, and red blood cell production

Potential Deficiencies: Depression, fatigue, insomnia, impaired
immunity, nerve pain, seasonal affective disorder (SAD),
seizures, skin rashes

Plant-Based Sources: Avocado, bananas, beans, cardamom,
chickpeas, onion, peanut, pistachio, potato, spinach,
sweet potato, sunflower seed, tarragon, turmeric

Vitamin B_9

AKA: Folate, folacin, folic acid

Functions in the Body: Growth and normal cell development;
decreased risks of heart disease, colon, and cervical
cancers

Potential Deficiencies: Anemia, birth defects (increased risk for
neural tube defects during pregnancy), cancer, depression, fatigue, heart disease, memory loss

Plant-Based Sources: Dark green leafy vegetables (e.g., kale,
spinach), onion, tarragon, turmeric

Nutrient Note: High folate intake may mask a B_{12} deficiency,
so it's important to have both micronutrient levels
screened in your bloodwork.

Most people can meet their daily micronutrient needs with
plant-based food sources and without the use of supplements.
The exception to this is vitamin B_{12}. Since vitamin B_{12} is found
in animal products, fortified foods or a supplement may be
necessary.

Vitamin B$_{12}$

AKA: Cobalamin, cyanocobalamin

Functions in the Body: Normal cognition and neurotransmit-
ter production, red blood cell formation, nerve function,
DNA production, cell metabolism

Potential Deficiencies: Anemia, depression, dizziness, fatigue,
insomnia, irritability, loss of appetite, mood changes,
neurological problems, "pins and needles" (extremities),
weakness

Plant-Based Sources: Soy (beans, tofu, tempeh, etc.), fortified
soy milk, fortified cereal

Vitamin C

AKA: Ascorbic acid, calcium ascorbate

Functions in the Body: Strengthens immunity; promotes
wound healing; decreases risk of heart disease, cancer,
cataracts, and memory loss

Potential Deficiencies: Scurvy (bleeding gums, bruising,
fatigue, rash, weakness)

Plant-Based Sources: Broccoli, brussels sprouts, cardamom,
chives, citrus fruits, collard greens, green pepper, kiwi,
melon, onion, papaya, paprika, strawberries, tarragon,
tomatoes, turmeric

Since these water-soluble vitamins lose the most micronutrients when cooked, your body's nutrient absorption will increase by eating the noted fruits, vegetables, herbs, and spices
raw when possible and safe to do so.

Fat-Soluble Vitamins

Unlike water-soluble vitamins, fat-soluble vitamins (vitamins
A, D, E, and K) are stored in the body's fatty tissues and liver

for up to six months, to be used as needed. Also unlike their water-soluble counterparts, fat-soluble vitamins retain substantially more micronutrients when cooked.

Plant-based food sources containing fat-soluble vitamins should be paired with other forms of healthy fats in order to increase bioavailability (to best dissolve the micronutrients and prepare them for absorption into the body). As you will see outlined by each micronutrient, fat-soluble foods containing vitamin A (squash, sweet potatoes, and carrots), vitamin D (mushrooms), vitamin E (asparagus, spinach, and swiss chard), and vitamin K (broccoli, kale, and spinach) are all absorbed better when eaten with one or two one-ounce portions of healthy fats (like avocado, mixed nuts, or olive oil).

Vitamin A

AKA: Retinol, beta-carotene (converts to vitamin A)

Functions in the Body: Immunity; lowers risk of certain cancers, heart disease, and cataracts; formation of soft tissue, mucous membranes, and skin; improves vision and eye health; bone and tooth formation

Potential Deficiencies: Dry eyes and skin, frequent infections (mild to severe), night blindness

Plant-Based Sources: Asparagus, beets, broccoli, cantaloupe, carrots, chard, chives, collard greens, dandelion, kale, paprika, pumpkin, spinach, squash, sweet potato, tarragon, tomato, turnip greens

Cooking Impact: Eating pumpkin and sweet potato with small amounts of "healthy" fat (like olive oil) will increase the body's absorption of beta-carotene.

Vitamin D

AKA: D$_3$, cholecalciferol

Functions in the Body: Bone health (assists in calcium absorption and deposit into bones), lowers risk for colon cancer and depression

Potential Deficiencies: Bone pain, fatigue, increased risk of heart disease, lowered immunity, mood changes, muscle aches / weakness, osteoporosis

Plant-Based Sources: Almonds, fortified soy, safflower oil, spinach, turmeric

Note: Ten to fifteen minutes of direct, unfiltered sunlight (not through a window) will also provide you with your necessary daily vitamin D requirements.

Vitamin E

AKA: D-alpha-tocopherol

Functions in the Body: Enhances immunity, prevents clotting in heart, lowers risk of heart disease and cancer

Potential Deficiencies: Nerve and muscle damage, muscle weakness, vision problems, weakened immunity, peripheral neuropathy

Plant-Based Sources: Almonds, asparagus, avocado, beet greens, collard greens, mangoes, peanuts, peanut butter, pumpkin, red bell pepper, spinach, safflower / soybean / sunflower oils, sunflower seeds, turmeric, wheat germ oil

Vitamin K

AKA: Phylloquinone

Functions in the Body: Blood clotting, bone and heart health

Potential Deficiencies: Impaired blood clotting, increased risk of heart disease, osteoporosis

Plant-Based Sources: Avocado, blueberries, broccoli, brussels sprouts, collard greens, figs, garden cress, green beans, kale, kiwi, mustard greens, parsley, prunes, soybeans, swiss chard, turmeric, turnip, urtica

Note: Individuals risk excess bleeding if taking blood thinners along with vitamin K and should consult with their healthcare providers about their dietary intake.

Minerals

Calcium

AKA: Calcium carbonate, calcium citrate

Functions in the Body: Aids in blood clotting, blood pressure regulation, muscle contraction, and neural transmission; lowers risk of osteoporosis

Potential Deficiencies: Brain fog, dizziness, fatigue, insomnia, irregular heartbeat, muscle cramps

Plant-Based Sources: Amaranth leaves*, black beans, cardamom, collard greens*, fortified orange juice, lamb's-quarters*, mustard seeds*, nettles*, nopales*, soy (fortified milk, tahini, tofu), spinach*, tarragon, turmeric

Cooking Note: Calcium-containing foods above marked with an asterisk (*) are absorbed better when cooked.

Iron

AKA: Ferrous fumarate, ferrous sulfate

Functions in the Body: Oxygen transportation in the red blood cells and muscle cells, neurological development, immune system and hormone synthesis

Potential Deficiencies: Pica (strange cravings to consume non-food items, such as dirt, clay, or paper), anemia (low red blood cell count), depression, pale skin, extreme fatigue, heart disease, weakness

Plant-Based Sources: Cardamom, leafy green vegetables, legumes, nuts, seaweed, seeds (pumpkin, sesame, squash), soybeans (natto, tempeh, tofu), spinach, tarragon, thyme, turmeric, whole grains

Cooking Notes: For additional iron, cook with cast-iron pans. Pair plant-based food sources containing both iron and vitamin C to boost absorption of both. Avoid simultaneous consumption of calcium and iron; avoid eating iron sources with tea, coffee, and/or calcium supplements (separate by two hours before and after eating). See cooking tips on page 146 for further details.

Magnesium

AKA: Magnesium citrate, magnesium gluconate, magnesium hydroxide, magnesium oxide

Functions in the Body: Anxiety, blood pressure regulation, bone formation and maintenance, heart function, muscle relaxation, nerve transmission, sleep, stress management

Potential Deficiencies: Depression, impaired sleep, insomnia

Plant-Based Sources: Bananas, cardamom, dark green leafy vegetables, legumes (beans and peas), nuts, soybeans, tarragon, turmeric, wheat germ, whole grains

Trace Minerals

Chromium

AKA: Chromium picolinate, chromium nicotinate

Functions in the Body: Carbohydrate metabolism and insulin action, glucose regulation, lowers cholesterol

Potential Deficiencies: Anxiety, glaucoma, increases diabetes risk, heart disease, skin conditions, muscle weakness

Plant-Based Sources: Brazil nuts, broccoli, grapes, onion, whole grain cereals, whole wheat products

Copper

AKA: Cupric oxide, copper gluconate, copper oxide, copper sulfate

Functions in the Body: Glucose regulation, heart and brain function, nerve transmission, red blood cell formation

Potential Deficiencies: Disrupted sleep patterns, early hair graying, fatigue, impaired immunity, neurological problems

Plant-Based Sources: Avocado, banana, green vegetables, potatoes, soybeans

Manganese

AKA: Manganese sulfate

Functions in the Body: Bone health, glucose regulation, metabolism, wound healing

Potential Deficiencies: Bone demineralization, impaired glucose tolerance, skin rash

Plant-Based Sources: Brown rice, black pepper, cardamom, hazelnuts, legumes (chickpeas, lentils, soybeans), oatmeal, onion, pecans, pumpkin seeds, spinach, tarragon, tofu, turmeric

Selenium

AKA: L-selenomethionine

Functions in the Body: Lowers risk of depression, heart disease, and rheumatoid arthritis

Potential Deficiencies: Brain fog, cardiomyopathy, depression, fatigue, hair loss, male and female infertility, weakened immune system

Plant-Based Sources: Baked beans, Brazil nuts, brown or white rice, oatmeal, tarragon, whole grain pasta, whole grain cereals and breads

Zinc

AKA: Zinc gluconate, zinc picolinate, zinc sulfate monohydrate

Functions in the Body: Enhances immunity, lowers depression risk, taste and smell sensitivity, wound healing

Potential Deficiencies: Cold symptoms, delayed wound healing, diarrhea, hair loss, rash, trouble concentrating, vision problems

Plant-Based Sources: Beans, cardamom, cashews, chervil, legumes (chickpeas, lentils), oregano, pumpkin seeds, thyme, turmeric, walnuts, water hyssop, whole grains

Cooking Note: Pair plant-based foods containing zinc (listed above) with those containing sulfur (such as garlic and onions) for increased absorption.

Cooking Tips for Increased Bioavailability of Plant-Based Food Sources

To review, water-soluble vitamins (B vitamins and vitamin C) lose the most micronutrients when cooked, and fat-soluble vitamins (A, D, E, K) lose the fewest. In terms of cooking methods, the most micronutrients are lost by boiling in water. For best bioavailability, eat most plant-based sources of water-soluble and heat-sensitive micronutrients in raw form.

To translate, water-soluble micronutrients (like vitamins B_1, folate, and vitamin C) are best eaten in raw form to maximize their absorption in the body. These include sunflower seeds, peas, beet greens, and brussels sprouts (vitamin B_1 sources); spinach, turnip greens, and broccoli (folate sources); and bell peppers, broccoli, and brussels sprouts (vitamin C sources).

Canned produce is often as nutritious as fresh, as canning occurs within hours of picking and keeps micronutrients (vitamins and minerals) intact.

Like most things in life, when it comes to cooking methods and plant-based micronutrients, it doesn't have to be all or nothing. I'll use spinach as a practical example. Raw spinach contains roughly three times more vitamin C than its boiled version. However, it's important to be practical and consider all factors, like quantity. For those of us inclined to eat spinach, it's a lot easier to eat five cups of cooked spinach than five cups of raw spinach. So it's fine to cook spinach at low heat without using excess water and losing the micronutrients we want. Cooking methods like microwaving, roasting, sautéing, or steaming offer a compromise.

Of course, in some cases, micronutrient bioavailability is increased when foods are cooked. The bioavailability of beta-carotene, found in most red, yellow, and orange plant-based foods (carrots, sweet potatoes, tomatoes), is significantly increased when cooked, as heat breaks down cellular walls within plants. Cooking also makes minerals (like calcium, iron, and magnesium) more bioavailable by decreasing oxalates, to which minerals may bind; limiting oxalates increases mineral absorption by the body.

For similar reasons, food preparation also makes a considerable difference in micronutrient content. Food prep basics can increase bioavailability of micronutrients in a number of ways. As with different forms of cooking, micronutrient absorption can be impacted by whether or not the foods containing them have been cut, crushed, chopped, or soaked prior to cooking. Cutting up and crushing foods will typically have a similar effect as breaking down cellular walls within plants and releasing micronutrients. For example, when onions and garlic are cut, chopped, and crushed, a sulfur-containing compound called **allicin** is produced. When eaten, allicin helps to form a chain of other protective compounds, but one side effect is its eye-watering effect. (Refrigerating the onion or other sulfur-containing food source for at least thirty minutes before cutting should help reduce the irritation.) Soaking whole grains, seeds, legumes (beans, peas, lentils), and some nuts for twenty-four hours has an impact on your micronutrient intake, as doing so will reduce phytate (phytic acid) content, which has been shown to interfere with calcium, iron, magnesium, and zinc absorption.

Pairing your plant-based foods may maximize micronutrient absorption in certain cases, just as keeping some food sources apart may do the same. To significantly increase iron absorption from plant-based sources, pair these foods with a source of vitamin C, which prompts the plant-based food to release the iron. Examples of iron sources paired with vitamin C include kale, lentils, spinach, and soybeans (sources of iron) coupled with lemon juice, orange slices, or strawberries (sources of vitamin C). In contrast, don't pair sources of iron with sources of calcium; wait at least two hours between ingesting them.

Storing your plant-based food sources correctly will also affect their micronutrient levels, which are primarily degraded by oxygen, light, and heat. To hold off degradation as long as possible, in the best interests of your nutrition and wallet, I suggest the following:

1. Refrigerate vegetables (except roots) until you use them.
2. Store fruits (including avocadoes and tomatoes, but not berries) out of direct light and at room temperature.
3. Squeeze lemon juice on any already prepped (cut or chopped) plant-based foods and place them an airtight container.
4. Chop up herbs to freeze with water in an ice cube tray (my favorite tip).

Believe it or not, my goal with this article was to inform while keeping things simple and sane. Some people can become obsessive with this topic, and I don't want you to be one of them. After reviewing the plant-based food sources mentioned in this article, I expect you could choose from the wide variety of colorful options available to you in your area and "eat the rainbow" daily, as most registered dietitians say. You don't need a spreadsheet to tell you that 70 percent of a micronutrient is better than 0 percent of nothing. It's always easier to focus on foods you tend to like, prepared in a manner you prefer, to increase your chances for successfully eating them. To get those five servings a day, your options include raw, lightly cooked, cooked, paired, unpaired, and various ways of storage. Check out the resources on the next page for further information, and leave the insanity to the professionals!

Resources

"Canned Food Facts." Canstruction. Accessed August 1, 2023. https://www.canstruction.org/canfoodfacts.

US Department of Agriculture. "What Is MyPlate?" MyPlate. Accessed July 30, 2023. https://www.myplate.gov/eat-healty/what-is-myplate.

US Department of Agriculture and US Department of Health and Human Services. "Dietary Guidelines for Americans, 2020–2025." 9th Edition. December 2020. https://www.dietaryguidelines.gov/resources/2020-2025-dietary-guidelines-online-materials.

"Vegetarian and Plant-Based." Academy of Nutrition and Dietetics. Accessed July 31, 2023. https://www.eatright.org/health/wellness/vegetarian-and-plant-based.

Delicious Energizing Herbal Food and Drinks

⚘ Holly Bellebuono ⚘

When I feel fatigued—flat-out tired, exhausted, or simply sad—plants often have the answer. Herbs are those wonderful friends who will give us a little pick-me-up when we need it. I've found that through the various stages of life I've lived—from raising children to now approaching menopause—herbal foods and drinks are the go-to for sustaining my energy in a steady, flavorful, and enjoyable way. They're safe, they're delicious, and they're generally easy to prepare.

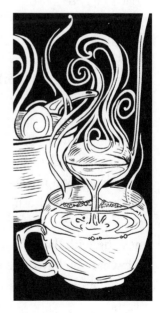

I advocate using nourishing herbs and tonics for energy rather than sports drinks that provide "punches" of caffeine but no long-term benefit. Cans of sugary, caffeine-spiked drinks will lead to drowsiness and also to a bizarre form of addiction. Herbs, on the other hand, provide a sustained feeling of contentment and energy because of their vitamins and minerals. Most of us don't think of stinging nettle (*Urtica dioica*) as an energy food and wouldn't group it in the same enlivening category as ginseng (*Panax ginseng*). But I've found that nettle is one of the most supportive herbs there is, and I use it as a foundational herb for energizing foods and drinks such as the ones that follow. Plus, it has a deep, resonant flavor that combines well with other herbs without overpowering a recipe.

Now that I've worked with edible and medicinal herbs for over three decades (since 1994), I've learned that energy comes in a wide range of forms. There's bouncy energy for getting chores done; there's steady energy for thinking and brainstorming. Energy can be sweet (like the gingerbread hot winter milk recipe on page 156) or it can be tangy (like the essential energy dressing on page 154, drizzled over cheese, potatoes, or fish). Energy is decidedly versatile—a variety of flavors, colors, textures, and scents makes for a lovely world to live in. Even gratitude is an energy. As herbalists and gardeners, we are so lucky to be able to get our hands and tastebuds on a wide variety of incredible plants—sampling, tasting, testing, and experimenting. The following recipes are meant to be "frittered" with until you find what resonates for you.

In these recipes, I've shared ways to include herbs whether they're growing fresh outside your door or they have been dried or frozen. Don't let the season keep you from experimenting with flavorful, nutritious herbs and spices for energy. Use what you have on hand without feeling the need to locate unusual ingredients; above all, enjoy the process and share the plants.

ᔈ Chia Seed Energy Balls

Many herbalists, including myself, love to use herbal powders and nut butters to make nourishing snacks. These little energy balls are held together with almond butter (or use any kind of thick nut or seed paste, such as peanut or sunflower) and chia seeds. Chia is now widely available, keeps well in the pantry, and has just enough crunch to give these balls texture. A few energy balls pair well with apple slices or a hard-boiled egg.

You will need:

- 1 cup almond butter (or any nut or seed butter, such as sunflower seed butter or tahini)
- 3–4 tablespoons chia seeds
- 3 tablespoons raw sunflower seeds
- ¼ cup ground flaxseed
- 1–2 tablespoons herbal powders: choose a mix from ginseng, eleuthero, ginger, peppermint, amla, nettle, spirulina, cinnamon, cardamom, or other powder of choice
- 2–4 teaspoons molasses or maple syrup
- ¼ teaspoon vanilla extract
- 2–4 teaspoons of cocoa powder (optional)
- 2–4 teaspoons additional chia seeds (optional)

In a medium bowl, stir together all the ingredients until well combined. Adjust for seasoning and texture: if the mixture is too gooey, add more flax, powder, or chia seeds. If it's too stiff, add more molasses or maple syrup. Using your fingers, roll the mixture into small balls, and then dredge each little ball onto a plate of the optional cocoa or chia seeds, if desired. To store the balls, layer them between sheets of wax paper in a storage container, seal tightly, and refrigerate for up to 7 days. Makes 20 balls, about 1¼ inches in diameter.

⤜ Essential Energy Dressing

This dressing is for so much more than salads; see the next page for serving ideas. Prepare this dressing in the summer or fall using fresh fruits, or make it in the winter from frozen berries, fruits, and dried herbs.

You will need:
- 1 quart white wine, white wine vinegar, or apple cider vinegar
- 1 cup fresh elderberries, or ½ cup dried
- 2 cups pitted fruit (choose from plums, peaches, mangoes), sliced
- 1 cup fresh or frozen cranberries or blueberries
- ½ cup total dried herbs such as nettle, hyssop, lemon balm, or alfalfa (optional)
- 1 cup raw cane sugar or honey (optional)

Gently warm the wine or vinegar in a large saucepan over medium-low heat. Place the herbs in a 1-quart glass canning jar and pour the warmed vinegar over them. Use a long-handled wooden spoon to release air bubbles and "smoosh" the fruit a bit. Cap tightly with a nonmetallic lid. Place the jar on a small dish to catch any liquid that may ooze out, and store it in a cupboard or other dark place for at least 2 weeks.

Strain the dressing through a cheesecloth. Return it to the saucepan and gently whisk the optional sugar or honey into the vinegar, gently reheating if necessary. Store the strained, infused vinegar in a clean, labeled jar or bottle, and use within 2 years.

Essential Energy Dressing Serving Ideas

- As an ice cream topping: gently reheat 1 cup of the dressing and add more sweetener if desired. Drizzle over vanilla ice cream or fruit sorbets.

- For brie and soft cheeses: gently reheat 1 cup of the dressing and stir in salt and pepper. Drizzle over soft cheese and serve with crackers or focaccia.

- For vegetables: gently reheat 1 cup of the dressing and stir in salt, pepper, and other herbs as desired, such as thyme or marjoram. I like to add a bit of butter or olive oil to the saucepan for a creamier sauce. Drizzle over roasted red peppers, asparagus, or roasted potatoes.

- For meat: gently reheat 1 cup of the dressing and stir in salt, pepper, and other herbs or spices, such as dill or fennel. I like to add a bit of butter or olive oil to the saucepan for a creamier sauce. Drizzle over sliced roasted chicken or fish.

Gingerbread Hot Winter Milk

Drink this soothing, fragrant hot milk when you need a warming pick-me-up on a cold day. Alongside a slice of freshly baked pumpkin bread, this aromatic beverage will soothe the soul. A bonus recipe for aromatic whipped cream follows and can top any special winter cake or pie. Start with a powder blend for flavoring.

≈ Gingerbread Powder Blend

2 teaspoons ground ginger

1 teaspoon ground cinnamon

1 teaspoon licorice root powder

To make the powder blend, stir together the spices in a small glass jar, then cap and label. Store on the countertop.

≈ Gingerbread Hot Winter Milk

2 cups fresh creamy oat milk or cow's milk

½–1 teaspoon gingerbread powder blend (see above)

2 cardamom pods

1 to 2 whole cloves

To make the hot herbal milk, pour the milk into a small saucepan over medium heat. Add the gingerbread powder blend, cardamom, and cloves. Heat until the milk scalds, just below the boiling point, about 5–8 minutes. Strain out the solids and pour the milk into 4 hot mugs. Serve alongside warm lemon scones, gingerbread, or pumpkin pie.

≈ Gingerbread-Scented Whipped Cream

2 cups cold heavy whipping cream

½–1 teaspoon gingerbread powder blend (see above)

1–2 teaspoons powdered sugar

1–2 teaspoons tapioca or arrowroot powder

1 teaspoon vanilla extract

To make the whipped cream, place the cold heavy whipping cream in a large, deep bowl. Add the gingerbread powder blend, sugar, tapioca or arrowroot powder, and vanilla extract. Using a strong whisk, whisk the mixture until soft peaks form. This is a workout! Keep going until the cream does not fall off the whisk when you pull it out, but instead forms a soft mound. Alternatively, use an electric handheld beater. Dollop the finished whipped cream over cakes, pies, berries, oatmeal, or hot cocoa.

Celebration Mulling Blend and Mulled Drinks

For an energizing treat with depth and pronounced flavor, make a mulling blend and use it with either red wine or apple cider. I love how the house smells so fragrant when this is cooking. This mulling blend uses traditional spices as well as unconventional herbs for flavor highlights. If you already have a store-bought mulling blend, feel free to add herbs to it. Use whatever you have on hand, and go easy on the cloves, as they are more powerful than you think!

⚘ Herbal Mulling Blend

5–6 whole black peppercorns

2–3 whole cloves

2 cardamom pods

1 whole allspice

1 (3-inch) cinnamon stick

Add the following if desired:

1 teaspoon dried chopped gingerroot

1 teaspoon dried lemon peel (diced, not granules)

1 teaspoon dried hibiscus flowers

1 teaspoon dried nettle leaves

Combine all the spices and herbs in a bowl. Use the scent to decide if you'd like to adjust quantities. Store in a tightly lidded jar and label it.

If your blends or dressings taste too strongly of clove after you've made them, adjust the flavoring with an herb that has the opposite flavor. For instance, while clove is bitter and strong, nettle and elderberry have depth and are not bitter. Reheat or reblend your recipe using nettle or elderberry if you find the clove is too much.

ᵅ Herbal Mulled Wine

1 jar herbal mulling blend (see page 157)

1 bottle red wine (preferably dry, nothing too expensive!)

2 tablespoons sugar

4–5 slices fresh orange (optional)

¼ cup fresh orange juice

Heat a skillet to medium and add the mulling blend from the jar. Stir until the mixture is fragrant, about 2 to 3 minutes. Don't let it burn! Remove from heat and scrape the mix onto a plate.

In a medium saucepan, combine the wine, mulling mixture, sugar, oranges, and orange juice. Use a tea bag if you wish to keep the spices in a bag; otherwise stir them into the wine loosely. Heat to a simmer (not a boil), then reduce heat and gently warm the wine for 30 minutes. Strain through a cheesecloth and serve in mugs or thick glasses.

✎ Herbal Mulled Apple Cider

    1 jar herbal mulling blend (see page 157)

    ½ gallon apple cider

    2 tablespoons sugar (optional)

    4–5 slices fresh orange (optional)

    ¼ cup fresh orange juice

It's optional to heat the spice mixture in this recipe, as the stronger flavor might overpower the apple cider. If you choose to heat it, heat a skillet to medium and add the mulling blend from the jar. Stir until the mixture is fragrant, about 2 to 3 minutes. Don't let it burn! Remove from heat and scrape the mix onto a plate.

The sugar is optional since the apple cider is naturally sweet. Otherwise, combine all the ingredients in a medium saucepan and bring to a simmer. Continue to heat uncovered for 25–30 minutes. Strain through a cheesecloth, taste for sweetness, and serve in mugs or thick glasses.

The Herbs You Really Need

❧ Bonnie Rose Weaver ❧

The herbs you really need are the ones you already have. Capitalism has tried to trick you into believing otherwise. The herbs you need are not expensive. They are not hard to find, they are not obscure or hard to pronounce. The herbs you need are the herbs already in your kitchen.

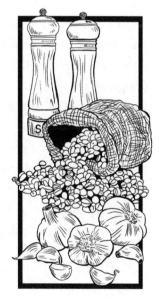

Take stock—what's in your spice cabinet? What herbs do you buy fresh at the farmers' market or grocery store? What is your favorite sprinkle on rice, chicken, or salad? What herbs do you long for and miss terribly when you are traveling or the pantry is running low?

Some of the most common herbs found in "a typical American kitchen" are coffee, salt, pepper, garlic, and parsley. At first glance, you may raise an eyebrow at the thought of these being anything more than a flavor enhancer or garnish.

Believe it or not, the more common and widespread an herb, the safer it is. By and large, these herbs are safe for kids and those who are pregnant, elderly, or chronically ill. They are safe enough to be incorporated into food, and yes, they are also medicinal. (Though please remember to consult a trusted healthcare provider with any questions when making changes to your diet or healthcare routine.)

All of the most common kitchen or culinary herbs you are familiar with for sprucing up a stir-fry, curry, salad, roast, sauce, or even a batch of cookies nudge the body in a particular direction toward balance or homeostasis. We call these **herbal actions**, which is a term that describes how the herb "works" in the body. For example, a familiar herbal action is anti-inflammatory. Turmeric (*Curcuma longa*) can reduce inflammation in the body, having particular importance for athletes and people with arthritis. Take note of the herbal actions peppered throughout the text to immerse yourself in the holistic function of your food.

If you want to be more thrifty, show off at a dinner party when the conversation lulls, or be prepared for a first-aid solution in a pinch, these basic remedies will surprise you. Prepare to fall in love with parsley and to never look at pepper the same way again. This is some basic-bitch shit that will make you absolutely love being basic. You're welcome.

Coffee (*Coffea,* *C. arabica,* and *C. canephora*)

Coffee? An herb?! What is an herb? you might ask. Depending on the context, there are different definitions. What's important here is that we are going to look at the medicinal qualities of a plant and the actions they take on the body.

Coffee is, for a great majority of the world, a favorite morning drink. The bean that greases the gears of productivity is best known for the phytochemical compound caffeine. What does caffeine do in the body? It makes our heart pump faster and, in a balanced dosage, can act as a cardiotonic. Too much, however, may leave you feeling anxious. An increased heart rate can take effect on how we move through the world; coffee can flip the switch on our reactions from parasympathetic (rest and digest) to the less desirable sympathetic (fight, flight, or freeze) states of being. Consider: How do you want to move through the world?

Caffeine also stimulates blood flow to the brain, acting as a brain stimulant, a balm for a case of the Mondays and the gas pedal of productivity for quicker and clearer thoughts. As a stimulant to the central nervous system, coffee can have a big effect on how we respond. Insomnia, stress, anxiety, and worry can all be exacerbated by the use of coffee. We might think that one cup of coffee in the morning has no effect on the quality of our sleep at night. However, we are not robots with an on/off switch. Everything in our bodies is connected!

Western science loves to pick apart and separate things, and we must not forget how interconnected and interdependent we are. The heart is a part of the cardiovascular system, and it is directly involved with all other body systems. Coffee takes noticeable effect on several other systems, including the nervous, digestive, respiratory, and lymphatic systems.

How? Coffee is **bitter**. The bitter principle states that any bitter flavor will stimulate all parts of the digestive system, including increasing salivation in the mouth, acid stimulation in the stomach and liver, and movement in the intestines. Just one sip of coffee can help relieve sluggish digestion and produce the long-awaited or ritualistic bowel movement.

As a bronchodilator, coffee can be used in a pinch for a person with labored breathing, due to asthma or a seasonal cold. As a diuretic, coffee can support a person who holds water in the body during PMS. This can look like swollen ankles or breast tenderness. Also an astringent, coffee supports the body to find balance with liquids. An unexpected bee sting can be soothed with a poultice of wet ground coffee directly on the affected skin.

Now that you are better acquainted with the medicinal qualities of coffee, you may reconsider when and in what dosage you want to incorporate the herb in your life. The beverage is so commonplace in our dominant culture that it can be hard to escape. If you are looking for a shift in your energy levels, consider choosing green tea or energizing with nettle tea first thing in the morning. This can help balance the ebb and flow of hyper energy, anxiety, and insomnia patterns for people wishing to get more or deeper sleep.

Your cup of joe might be a lot more potent than you previously thought!

Salt (Sodium Chloride, NaCl)

Salt, an incredibly useful crystal, is a common and favorite ingredient to increase the flavor in food. How lovely to let it linger on one's tongue, as this rock is cleansing and clearing.

A dip in the big blue is refreshing, rejuvenating, clearing, and centering. Sitting and watching the waves of salt water move with the rhythm of the moon is beneficial to the body and mind. The salt in ocean water exposes a person to negative ions. Salt lamps offer a similar effect to reduce the harmful elctromagnetic fields of computers and other electronics.

Salt is critical in the fermentation process for sauerkraut and kimchi, as it draws out the moisture of cabbage and other crunchy veggies to produce a salty brine, which then preserves the food for many months. The result is a belly-supporting snack filled with probiotics to support our microbiome, a critical component of our immune system linked to how we think.

As an antibacterial, salt acts as a hypertonic, wicking moisture to reduce or prevent bacteria. In this way, warm salt water is an incredible healer in cleaning wounds and a gentle flush for clearing congested sinuses. Use in a bath or foot bath with a warming herb like pepper, mustard powder, or rosemary to cleanse and warm the body on a chilly day.

Feeling dehydrated? Mix a couple of pinches of salt in water with a spoonful of honey and a squeeze of lemon to make an easy electrolyte tonic.

Sweat, tears, or the sea—salt is a profound healer.

Black Pepper (*Piper nigrum*)

Pepper, how I love thee. Warming and activating this herb gives direction to others. When we add pepper to food, we are better able to digest and assimilate a meal. This is due to the carminative quality of the aromatic peppercorn. A **carminative** is a substance, in this case a plant, that supports the body to improve digestion and absorption of nutrients into the body. This means gas up or down, digestive pain, discomfort, diarrhea, and constipation are reduced. Black pepper is also a **harmonizer**. When blended with other herbs in an herbal formula, pepper acts in support of other herbs and directs the herb, like turmeric, to areas of the body where the medicine is needed most.

I want to make sure you are sitting down for this next one: black peppercorns are the stone fruit of a flowering vine. And this fruit is an unsuspecting source for phytocannabinoids, along with sunflower, echinacea, cacao, and kava! That's right, plants that interact with your cannabinoid receptors, just like cannabis, are is present in every grocery store, restaurant, and likely your very own kitchen. This means a few grinds of pepper may subtly stimulate the endocannabinoid system, offering calming and anti-inflammatory effects throughout the body.

The remedy can also be applied externally. Infused oil of pepper can warm the body for someone who runs cold, can be applied to the chest to expel a cold, or can be added to a salad dressing for increased medicinal benefit. Black pepper increases circulation, acts as a mild expectorant on the lungs, and warms the body. Note: be sure to avoid delicate areas when using pepper-infused oil.

Any herb with strong aromatic scent, especially where an essential oil can be extracted, holds antibacterial properties. On a physical level, these herbs protect us from harmful bacteria, and on an energetic level, we are also protected.

Pepper reminds us that herbs stay fresher and more potent if they are kept longer in a more whole form. For example, you may know that pepper is found on occasion as a black-and-white powder, while other times it is found as a small black ball. Think of the flavor difference of preground pepper versus when pepper is freshly ground from a pepper mill. The whole corn is able to maintain the active compounds longer and, therefore, able to deliver on flavor and medicinal quality much longer.

Common and abundant, pepper can be reached for when needing warmth or protection.

Garlic (*Allium sativum*)

Garlic is one of the herbs we often keep around that truly tastes and smells medicinal. It's a supreme ingredient in the age-old remedy of fire cider, which is an immune tonic staple. Many recipes for fire cider can be found online. The one I keep in my head is as follows:

1. Chop onion, garlic, horseradish, ginger, hot peppers, rosemary, and thyme in any amount.
2. Place the herbs to fit neatly in a clean mason jar of any size and cover the herbs with apple cider vinegar. Affix a nonmetal lid and let sit for 1 week to 3 months.
3. Strain with a fine cloth or strainer. Use the fire cider as a daily tonic in winter months or apply to food as desired. Take 30–90 drops 1–3 times per day as needed.

Garlic may act as a powerful antiviral, meaning that it can support the body's function of addressing a virus. Compared to cooked or dried garlic, fresh garlic provides the highest medicinal dosage, so while the delicious aroma can add to a sauce or stir-fry, the medicinal qualities are not so present. A favorite way to utilize the medicinal qualities of garlic is to mince a clove and add the herb to a spoonful of honey or nut butter. Almond butter is a personal favorite choice for flavor. It is a best practice to allow the minced garlic to sit for ten minutes before eating to allow enzymes in the herb to be exposed to oxygen and deliver a more potent medicine.

Garlic is known as a powerful antifungal. Once upon a time, I struggled with chronic yeast infections and a classic standby solution is a garlic suppository. Peel a clove with care, being mindful not to pierce or nick the clove. Insert it into the vaginal canal to allow a powerful antifungal "aromatherapy" to activate in the body as a possible cheap, easy, and DIY antifungal remedy.

The part of the plant we use is the bulb. Garlic bulb has an affinity for the lungs and is known as an expectorant, which is a substance that supports the movement and release of mucus in the lungs. As a hypotensive, garlic can help lower blood pressure. It is gently toning to the heart and is a plant that brings warmth to the body overall.

Use garlic to protect yourself from vampires. Perhaps this old adage is allegory for the way garlic protects us from bacteria, virus, or fungus. For all these reasons and more, it's not uncommon to find a clove or two of garlic in the bottom of my backpack for easy access and frequent use.

Parsley (*Petroselinum crispum*)

Has any other herb been so incredibly overlooked as parsley? Often thought of as a garnish, it's somehow inherently unsexy, yet I have to say it's an herb I get excited about. When I'm at the market and I see a particularly bushy bunch of flat-leaf parsley, I get a little turned on.

Parsley is considered a nutritive tonic, as it is high in vitamins A and C, iron, calcium, magnesium, and chlorophyll. Aside from it being a lovely way to prevent scurvy on a long voyage at sea, the fresh leaf can be used as a substitution for basil in pesto. One may consider a blend of parsley and basil, kale, cilantro, or dill or let parsley shine on its own. A delicious quick dinner, parsley pesto preserves a large market haul for a nutritious weeknight dinner.

Parsley is little-known as an emmenagogue or abortifacient. This is due to the high concentration of vitamin C found in the leaves of this plant. A high dose of parsley, along with other herbs, has historically been used as a covert at-home remedy to support the body naturally releasing the contents of the womb.

Easy to grow from seed or starts, parsley is a welcome member of a window box garden, pots, or other small-scale culinary home gardens. Use it as a pop of flavor in salads or add it to a fruit salad, smoothie, or infused "spa" water when you have this friend on hand. Due to a drop in flavor and thus potency, parsley is not recommended as a dried herb.

With so many beneficial properties, including as an antiinflammatory and antioxidant, instead of buying multivitamins, try parsley!

In conclusion, medicine is all around us. In our kitchens, grocery stores, and farmers' markets, there are herbal medicines hiding under our noses. The first step is to redefine what we call medicine; we must see food and medicine as a spectrum in which all plants belong. From there, we start to see and use plants as active players in our pursuit for well-being. Whether you're experienced or new to the herb world, the herbs you already have are the herbs you absolutely need.

A Brief Intro to Afrobotany

⪼ Iya Angelique "Sobande" Greer ⪻

Long before European colonization, Africans viewed the natural environment with the highest reverence. Africans understood the metaphysical forces of nature. They understood its power and sought to live in alignment with absolute truth with it. This included but was not limited to a clear understanding of the healing power of plants.

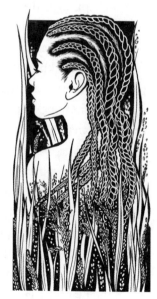

Africans specifically were targeted for agricultural slavery because their knowledge and experience were better suited to farming in the neotropical climates in the Americas than Europeans'. "In this way, their knowledge of plants—as well as their forced labor—made them vital to the success of the colonies," explains Alyson Morgan of the Herbal Academy. Africans' knowledge was both treasured and feared.

Traditions and philosophies centered around this mindset have been enforced and perpetuated in Western herbalism since the arrival of the first enslaved people in the Americas. Africans in the Americas owe their ability to adapt to these new lands to their ingenuity, determination, and familiarity with tropics, because they originated from similar regions in Africa. Enslaved people were able to blend old plant medicine knowledge with the terrain of their captors. They became popular medicine people along with the Indigenous tribes of the area. This medicine was highly regarded from New England to Brazil. Thus, early African American herbalism was based on a relationship and connection to the land.

They were, however, able to bring seeds of their local flora with them, such as by hiding them in hair. Cultural songs and stories kept alive the traditions for growing and using these plants. This knowledge hybridized with their experiences on plantations in the Americas, creating the foundation for the afrobotany we know today. "Much of the herbal knowledge gained in America came from direct connection, necessary learning, and the use of plants foraged in the woods, forests, and wetlands that provided a refuge from enslavement on plantations. For enslaved Africans and their descendants, herbalism and spiritual nourishment were intertwined. Plants supported their endurance and resilience in the face of enslavement," writes Morgan.

As their access to medical care was limited, herbalism offered a healing balm and empowerment. No matter where African people were transported on the planet, they incorporated the plants of land, the spirit of their collective ancestors, and their memories of their homeland into their everyday lives for health, wealth, and spirituality.

Many new or modified herbal traditions arose within Black communities in North America. These traditions were most celebrated, documented, and depended upon in the Southeast, where slavery was most concentrated. Typical elements included a combination of African, European, and Indigenous healing modalities, medicinal herbs, spiritual practices, and folklore. Voodoo, Ifá, and Santería are examples of this fusion whose practice is generally focused in the Caribbean, Louisiana, and other parts of the Deep South. Santería and Ifá are branches of the traditional religion of the Yoruba people from Nigeria that merged with Catholicism as a means of survival. Thus, the customary African gods are addressed under the names of Catholic saints.

African American Herbalism Today

The use of herbal remedies dwindled toward the end of the nineteenth century due to the rise of synthetic chemistry. We are seeing an enormous resurgence in plant medicines over the past twenty years, and herbalism in particular is resurfacing like never before in Black and Brown communities in America. The history and legacy of these practices are being honored, finding their place in our everyday lives to heal our minds, bodies, and spirits. Plants are part and parcel of our spiritual cosmology and form the truest meaning of what we call "holistic medicine." When we fail to acknowledge and honor the roots of this science, we fail humanity. And here in America, when we steal someone else's magic and discard the source . . . we fail humanity.

I was formally trained in herbalism by my great-grand-mother through the art of storytelling, hands-on kitchen work, and learning not to fear dirt.

My great-grandmother gave me the gift of silence. And knowing how to watch for signs.

My great-grandmother taught me how to pray and use my love to transform, transmit, and inspire a movement.

My great-grandmother taught me how to produce beautiful products and how to teach my children.

My great-grandmother taught me how to make something from nothing and how to embrace those who will never treat you right.

I practice herbalism every day of my life. Reconnecting and remembering the power of an ancient people who made mountains from ant hills. So it is my honor to be of service to my community.

Herbalism is a part of my everyday lifestyle. It is who I am at the core of my being. Herbalism is a force of nature that allows me to reconnect on a cellular level to the DNA of my ancestors, through song, meditation, chant, prayer, and community.

So I ask, as you move forward in your studies, teaching, training, sharing, exploring, visiting, and learning, please remember that it is imperative that healing hubs, centers, schools, conferences, workshops, apprenticeship programs, and those offering information in this field be open to the vast amount of knowledge and those who have access to it. If organizations never allow new faces of Black and Brown hues who represent the knowledge of their people, experiences, and cultures to share their history, it easily becomes lost, abandoned, and misconstrued.

This is a mere glimpse into my history as a descendant of enslaved Africans in America and a fraction of the magic we have poured into this country by force and choice.

It's time to decolonize the herbalism and holistic health movement—there is a place at the healing tree for all of us.

Resources

For more information on the history of afrobotany and decolonizing herbalism, check out these resources:

Morgan, Alyson. "Roots of African American Herbalism: Herbal Use by Enslaved Africans." Herbal Academy. August 18, 2020. https://theherbalacademy.com/african-american-herbalism-history/.

Penniman, Leah. *Farming While Black: Soul Fire Farm's Practical Guide to Liberation on the Land.* White River Junction, VT: Chelsea Green Publishing, 2018.

Ward, Priscilla. "Decolonizing Alternative Medicine: The Herbalism and Ecology of the African Diaspora." Healthline. August 16, 2021. https://www.healthline.com/health/decolonizing-alternative-medicine-uplifting-black-agro-ecological-traditions.

DIY
and
Crafts

Creating a Water Feature, One Pot at a Time

✺ JD Walker ✺

One of my earliest memories of my grandmother's landscape was the cement pond she built in her backyard. Readers of a certain age (or those raised on television reruns) will get the reference to a "cement pond." It was a running gag on the old show *The Beverly Hillbillies* (1962–71).

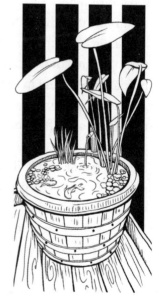

The show revolved around the humorous culture clash between a family of Missouri hill people (the Clampetts) who struck it rich after accidentally discovering oil on their property and the people they ran into when they moved to a mansion in Beverly Hills. The swimming pool behind the mansion was always referred to as a cement pond. Grandma loved the show.

Naturally, she had to have a cement pond of her own. Grandma constructed her pond by digging a six-by-four-foot hole in the ground roughly eighteen inches deep and lining it with concrete. She never set plants in it, but she was very fond of the goldfish she installed there.

As delightful as having a water feature might be, digging a pit for one might be a bit more than most homeowners would like to tackle. It might be entirely out of the question for those who rent! Fortunately, you don't need to go to that much trouble. All you need is a container, a good spot to set it, some water, and some imagination.

Location

Most gardeners will likely want their water feature located as close to their outdoor living area as possible. This could be on a patio or a deck or just somewhere in the landscape close to a comfortable chair. But they might be concerned about the availability of sunlight for their pond. After all, as we drive through the countryside, most of the ponds constructed by humans are sitting in the middle of a grazing area in full sun.

Farmers in my area have told me there was a conservation program after the Great Depression to encourage soil conservation by terracing the land and constructing ponds to control water and soil runoff. Having a water source in full sun is great for the cattle and horses but not necessary for a well-developed water container garden.

As little as three to four hours of direct sunlight will work well for most water plants. Six to eight hours might be needed if you intend to install tropical flowering water-loving plants. But too much sun could be a problem if you want fish in your water feature. The feature could overheat, killing the aquatic life.

Container

Now the fun begins—picking a container. Honestly, you can create a water feature in a container that only holds one gallon of water. It will not be big enough for most plants or more than one small fish. But if all you want is a spot of water with a little fountain and some floating plants, there is nothing wrong with that.

For more visual appeal, selecting a container that can hold five or more gallons is a good idea. Garden centers frequently carry whiskey barrels that have been cut in half that make excellent water garden containers. The shops also have plenty of decorative ceramic and clay pots. Don't forget that large metal or plastic pots and buckets can also be repurposed. Anyone who gardens probably has a spare ten-plus gallon container or two somewhere in the back of the garden shed.

The type of container is up to you. Many years ago, I took an old wheelbarrow that had seen better days, removed the wheel and handles, and sunk it into the ground outside the front room window. Because I used a liner, I could have just as easily left the wheelbarrow above ground and surrounded it with rocks.

There is one caveat. One gallon of water weighs just over eight pounds. A five-gallon container filled with water will weigh over forty pounds, and so on. Make sure your deck or porch will be able to hold the weight before you begin. Also, make certain you pick the right spot. Moving your water garden after it is established will be very difficult.

A five-gallon bucket or solid container will probably not need a liner. A whiskey barrel, an empty plant pot, or a repurposed container like my wheelbarrow bed definitely will. These are easy to install and will just need to be secured around the lip of the container to keep the liner from slipping. An inch of gravel at the bottom is a nice touch but not necessary.

You might wonder if you could just line your container with plastic sheeting. Yes, you can. However, the plastic will tend to degrade over the season and will have to be replaced for the next growing season. A rubberized liner specifically made for water features is more expensive, but it will last many years before needing to be replaced.

A filtration system is not necessary. Over time, your water feature will develop its own little ecosystem that will integrate plants and any aquatic life you install. A fountain is also not necessary. However, dancing waters lend a lot of character to a water feature. The water movement will also aerate the garden and help keep mosquito populations at bay.

Once filled, plants can be installed in your water garden immediately. You should wait three days before adding fish to allow the temperature and chemicals in the water to stabilize.

Plants

The possibility for plants in a water garden is extensive. When you design your garden, use the same tips that are employed for any patio container garden. Try to include plants of varying heights and textures to create the most interest. Tie everything together with low-growing or floater plants to complete your creation.

For vertical interest, consider a member of the iris family. A bog garden near me has an impressive collection of Louisiana irises (*Iris* spp.). Another popular member of the iris family is the yellow flag iris (*Iris pseudacorus*). Both have long, thick, grass-like foliage. They flower in late spring to early summer.

Another tall-grower is the exotic papyrus plant (*Cyperus papyrus*). While it doesn't have a very conspicuous flower, the umbel of greenish flowers that burst forth in summer provides a striking and long-lasting feature.

Other tall plants include rushes (*Juncus*), sedges (*Carex*), sweet flag (*Acorus calamus*), and even that summertime favorite, the canna lily. Cannas will give your garden a lush, broad-leafed contrast to the narrow leaves of plants discussed above. Just be sure to look for the aquatic canna lily (*Canna* 'Erebus').

Floaters are just what the name implies—they float on the surface of the water. Some hug the water's surface, like duckweed (*Lemna minor*) or azolla (*Azolla*). They look like you cast small-leaf foliage from a nearby bush on the water. Other floaters like parrot's feather (*Myriophyllum aquaticum*) and water hyacinth (*Pontederia crassipes*) grow to a height of three to twelve inches, completing the structural interest of your water garden.

Of course, most people want to know about growing water lilies (*Nymphaea*) or lotuses (*Nelumbo*) in a water feature. If you want to grow the hardy varieties, it is not too hard. In colder hardiness zones, tropical water lilies and lotuses will require special care to overwinter them in the coldest months.

First, the growing requirements. The floaters discussed above float on the water's surface. They are generally annuals that will need to be composted or otherwise disposed of in the winter. Please do not take these plants to a local water feature like a lake or stream. Some water plants are considered invasive in the wild.

The plants used for vertical accents are submerged. That means the pot and plant are sunk just below the water's surface.

Use a brick or overturned pot to get the right height for the plant. As long as your water garden will not freeze solid over the winter months, they will likely survive in place.

Water lilies and lotuses are sunk. The plant must be set at least six inches below the water's surface. If your water garden container is deep enough, you can actually fill the bottom of it with six to eight inches of soil to nest the container in. If you don't want to fill your container with soil, you will need to weigh the pot down with enough rocks to keep the plant from floating to the surface.

Hardy varieties of water lilies and lotuses should be able to overwinter in place. In plant zones above zone 7, where the water garden is likely to freeze over (or maybe freeze solid!), tropical varieties of these plants will need to be lifted from the water garden and stored in a dark spot where the temperature will not fall below 40 degrees Fahrenheit.

To Fish or Not to Fish

A water garden, even a well-designed one with plenty of plants, just begs for aquatic life. Fish have the added advantages of keeping mosquitoes out and controlling algae growth. Goldfish are the gold standard in a water feature. You don't have to settle for gold. Fancy goldfish can also be yellow, mottled, or black. You can even get those varieties called orandas that frankly creep me out with their bizarre "hoods" and bright colors. They look like someone crossed a fish with a Klingon, but if that makes you happy, go for it.

Minnows and guppies can also be put in a water garden but may need to be brought indoors over the winter. You should check with your local supplier about the recommendations for your area. In most areas, goldfish will survive in place over the winter without much trouble. Koi are great but require a large, deep pond to do well.

The general guideline is to install one fish per square foot of surface water. In my wheelbarrow water garden, I could technically have up to six fish (surface area roughly two by three feet). Any more than that can overwhelm the water feature's ecosystem, causing the fish to die off.

If you can't make your mind up about whether to have fish or not, don't worry. The local wildlife will soon discover your water feature. It is likely to become a favorite watering hole for birds, butterflies, dragonflies, and other insects. My pond draws toads, skinks, and lizards that are fun to watch as they sunbathe on the rocks surrounding the feature. The toads do lay eggs in the pond, but the resident goldfish usually take care of most of them. Only a few escape to become the next generation.

Conclusion

Fortunately, once established, a water garden doesn't need a lot of upkeep. Be sure to keep falling leaves out of the container in autumn. If summer in your area is especially hot or dry, you may need to add water to the feature from time to time.

Other than that, all you need is a chair, a cold beverage, and maybe a good book, and you will be all set for the season as you enjoy the pleasure of your own container water garden.

Resources

"Constructing and Caring for Container Water Gardens." University of Illinois Extension. Accessed August 29, 2023. https://web.extension.illinois.edu/containergardening/water_planting.cfm.

"How to Create a Mini Pond." The Wildlife Trusts. Accessed August 29, 2023. https://www.wildlifetrusts.org/actions/how-create-mini-pond.

How to Make a Herbarium Like Emily Dickinson

❧ Diana Rajchel ❧

A herbarium takes the botanical art of pressed flowers and scrapbooking and combines it with the community connection of contributing to scientific and historical records. Emily Dickinson herself kept one.

A herbarium was a book of herbs pressed on paper, complete with scientific notes. Often it tracked such data as where certain species grew and what chemicals they contained, and it came in handy for identification, whether for harvesting or foraging. Herbariums became popular with teen girls in the 1840s, likely because they provided a socially acceptable way to explore science—a field that at the time barred women—under the guise of art and expression.

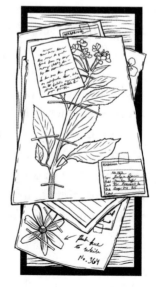

Dickinson's collection was a prolific 424 samples, now archived and made digitally available at the Harvard University library.

During the Victorian era, everything had rules—and Dickinson, much as she did in her literary aspect, broke them immediately. In traditional form, herbariums consisted of only local flowers, native to the collector's immediate environment. Pages contained notes regarding where archivists gathered the flowers, the Latin and common names, and the flower itself. Our rebel Emily opened her herbarium with tropical jasmine flower. She then conformed a bit, gathering flowers such as violets, rhododendrons, and other items that grew in her family's garden or near her home. Her herbarium is arranged with the deliberate symmetry and simplicity later found in her poems.

Outside of occasional unusual inclusions, her herbarium is artfully arranged, labeled, and simple. The samples she took remain valuable tools in scientific research because they allow botanists to identify how plants change where they grow, how leaves and flowers look, and what plants they grow beside throughout history. If you make a herbarium, you are making something artful and lovely. If you choose to label it in the traditional manner, this also preserves valuable information for future generations.

While the process of making a herbarium isn't difficult, it can be time-consuming. Depending on what archival tools you use, it can also get expensive. Decide before you begin how large of a record you want to create and how much you want to invest in the archival process.

Collection Process

You will need:

Notebook

Wax or parchment paper

Scissors

Trowel

Scotch tape (optional)

Before you head out to gather herbs, load up your collection basket: make sure you have garden gloves, a pair of scissors, a decent plant identification smartphone app or Audubon plant guide, any cultural items you may need to honor the plants you forage (such as offerings of tobacco or water), and a basket to gather the plants without squishing them. Goodwill and secondhand decor shops offer an abundance of baskets at any time of year, so no need to worry about the season in which you gather.

Because you won't be using these herbs for ingestion, public spaces with wild plants such as roadsides and parking lots are good places to gather samples. For instance, driving through my town in southwest Michigan, I can easily identify chicory, Queen Anne's lace, and dandelions cropping up in easements and at the edge of parking lots. All of these make lovely pressed flowers and are common enough not to cause a shortage in my area.

I do have to take safety into account, thus the need for the plant identification tools. Queen Anne's lace exemplifies one of the dangers of plant foraging for any purpose: as a member of the wild carrot family, it strongly resembles poison hemlock. While it grows shorter than hemlocks and is perfectly safe, an inexperienced plant collector can easily mistake the hemlock for the lace with results ranging from the uncomfortable (rashes, itching) to the fatal. Don't just find a pretty flower and pluck it. Ensure you use a good-quality plant identification app and a field or foraging guide to know, absolutely, the plant's identity. Do not collect anything if you are not 100 percent sure of what it is! You can always take a photo to share with people in plant identification forums and also run an image search with your phone.

In the interest of leaving plants to reproduce, and for other foragers, only take one plant from any location at a time. If you want a traditional-look herbarium, you may need to dig out the entire plant so that someone flipping through your book can also see the roots. If you want something that has more of a pressed-flowers scrapbook feel, you can opt only to take the blossom or cut at the stem, leaving the roots a chance to repropagate.

As you collect, write down the date, the name of the plant, the Latin name, and any identifiable plants growing nearby. For example, if you collect spring violets, you might make an entry like this:

April 7, 2026—common violet, Latin name *Viola sororia*

Found in the easement across the sidewalk from my neighbor's front yard, growing next to a hearty dandelion and bittercress. Found fresh earthworms floating up from the recent rain beside the sample, and a rabbit dashed across the street as I wrote.

Gently tear off a parchment or wax paper, fold it over your plant sample, and tape the outer edges closed. Repeat until you have gathered to your heart's desire.

Pressing Process

You will need:

Flower press or 2 large, thick books such as dictionaries or old encyclopedias

Flowers

The wax or parchment paper they are already folded into

The notebook with your identification comments

For those without the patience to wait at least 7 days, craft stores now carry flower presses, which come with features that allow you to dry the plant in the microwave! If you plan to invest in making many herbariums, or one large one, definitely consider purchasing one. I lean old-school and like the challenge of using what I have as much as possible. I enjoy finding reuses for big old books I buy at library book sales. For the low-tech version of flower pressing, choose a page in your large book, slide the paper with your plant sample inside, and tape the description from your notebook on top of the waxed or parchment paper. When you have all your plants lined up inside the book, close the book, pick a place shielded from heat and direct light, stack 3 or 4 other large books on top of it, and leave it for at least a week. I prefer to press flowers from season to season, so I retrieve mine after three to four months.

If you have concerns about the plant releasing too much moisture, open up the parchment or wax paper and fold some facial tissue or tissue paper around it before refolding the outer paper. I haven't found this a serious problem, but I'm also not using books I intend to reread someday.

Mounting Process

A note before you mount: If you intend to donate your herbarium to a scientific library, check with the organization about their archival requirements. Many research centers require that biological items use specific paper, adhesive, and preservatives. If you are making your own for fun, work with what you can afford and what is on hand. What I suggest here is intended for optimal results on a project intended for home, family, and friends.

You will need:

> PVA glue (also known as white, wood, or carpenter's glue)
>
> Your pressed flowers
>
> Heavy paper, preferably cardstock. You can potentially recycle greeting cards for this unless you want a much larger specimen book.
>
> Sleeve protectors (Acid-free paper and protectors are recommended.)

Take the cardstock you want to affix your flower to and give it a swipe of glue. Because I know some will hesitate, white glue dries transparent! It's okay to spread it around on your page!

Fix your plant to the glue. Next, write the identifying information on the page, or glue it from a separate scrap of paper. You can take the opportunity to add calligraphy, stamps, art, embossing, or other creative expression for any personal pages and notes. When it's dry, slip the page inside the sheet protector.

You may want to place the page inside a book again and press for a 1–2 extra days to ensure everything dries flat. I sometimes slip my pages between cardboard pieces cut from cereal boxes to help the plant redry flat after its exposure to the initially moist glue.

After 1–2 days of extra flat time, you're done! You've made your herbarium page!

After you have enough herbarium pages, you may choose to stitch a cover (again, cereal boxes make lovely book bases that you can decorate how you wish), or you can slip yours in a 3-ring binder. I prefer the 3-ring binder for herbariums intended to grow over years.

———

Dickinson lived when women could not participate in scientific study; what they were allowed to learn was either practical to the household or meant to make them more decorative and entertaining. Keeping a herbarium was a subversive act, an artistic, socially acceptable way for women to participate in scientific research. It presented a class of heavily restricted people a way of expressing emotion, through Victorian flower code, and ways of participating in an otherwise locked and restrictive world.

Nowadays, people of any persuasion can pursue science, poetry, or both, free from the need for socially acceptable subterfuge. Yet the appeal of such projects lives on. A herbarium is one of the more affordable and accessible ways to participate in furthering research and helping us understand the environment that we must steward. Even better, with the resurgence of interest in foraging, we now have more reason than ever to make personal herbariums—for reference, knowledge sharing, creative expression, and the sheer joy of natural beauty.

Resources

"Dickinson, Emily, 1830–1886. Herbarium, circa 1839–1846." Houghton Library, Harvard University. Accessed July 14, 2023. https://iiif.lib.harvard.edu/manifests/view/drs:4184689$1i.

Frank, Marc S. "What Is a Herbarium?" Florida Museum, University of Florida. December 22, 2016. https://www.floridamuseum.ufl.edu/science/what-is-a-herbarium/.

Grace. "An Easy Practical Way to Store Pressed Flowers." *Gardening-4Joy* (blog), September 2, 2022. https://www.gardening4joy.com/an-easy-practical-way-to-store-dried-pressed-flowers/.

Herb Society of America. "The Use and Methods of Making a Herbarium/Plant Specimens." Rev. ed. Kirtland, OH: Herb Society of America, 2005. https://www.herbsociety.org/file_download/inline/2c81731f-ecd5-4f5d-a142-666830a89ed2.

"Make Your Own Herbarium Specimens." School of Biosciences, University of Melbourne. 2018. https://biosciences.unimelb.edu.au/__data/assets/pdf_file/0010/2237788/MELU_MakeYourOwnHerb_Specimen_Dec18.pdf.

Popova, Maria. "Emily Dickinson's Herbarium: A Forgotten Treasure at the Intersection of Science and Poetry." *The Marginalian* (blog), May 5, 2017. https://www.themarginalian.org/2017/05/23/emily-dickinson-herbarium/.

Aromatic Fires

➢ Natalie Zaman ➢

O f all our senses, smell is the most powerful when it comes to conjuring memories. I know the "scent" of a museum or library (ah, old books!); the odorous, rubber scent of tires and the odd sweetness of gasoline; the damp earthiness that presages rain; and the smoky scent of wood burning.

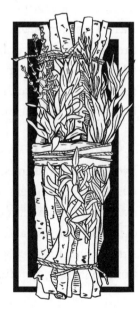

There's nothing quite like the smell of a wood fire (a planned one, of course!). There's something about the scent of wood smoke that is both outdoors and indoors. It evokes (for me) feelings of comfort and coziness. It triggers the notion, no matter what the season, that autumn, my favorite season, is not that far off. It brings me back decades: suddenly I'm seven years old again and toasting marshmallows for s'mores on the pebbly shores of Keuka Lake in upstate New York. Feeling heat on my face, streaming from a great blaze at a fall birthday party after a nighttime hayride through corn fields. Standing in front of the fireplace at my aunt's house on Christmas Eve—growing up in apartments, a fireplace was a real luxury.

All the fires I've just described smelled, as I recall, much the same, and what I thought all fires should smell like. So I was surprised one year to encounter an unfamiliar fire scent.

We were in Delray Beach in Florida and had the good fortune to spend a few nights at the Colony Hotel, a candy-colored art deco affair with a lobby straight out of an Old Hollywood movie from the 1930s. But what captured me the moment we breezed in wasn't the visual, but the scent of a wood fire burning in the fireplace. It was pungent and sweet, even incense-y. They were burning piñon logs. The word *piñon* conjured other memories, literary ones, as I recalled the Willa Cather novel *Death Comes for the Archbishop* that I'd read in college. That was the first time I'd ever heard of piñon logs, but I'd never actually experienced them. And here I was in this beautiful hotel, recalling all of these things . . . it was a spiritual moment. That is how important scent is.

Crafting Scented Logs and Kindling Bundles

I've always loved loose incense with large chunks of resins, whole leaves, flowers, needles, seeds, and pods. Blending my own incenses taught me new ways to unearth and create memories through fire and scent. Each season has its own special smells, and for each person, scents bring up different reactions, olfactory, emotional, and physical. Bonfires are for any season, and combinations of woods, herbs, and flowers serve to recall memories as well as create them.

Creating combinations of "ingredients" for scented fires is like the perfumer's art: **top notes** are immediate, what you smell even before the log or kindling bundle is burned. Some woods will definitely have a strong scent, but most of the top notes will come from dried herbs and flowers. **Heart or middle notes** come next. Crushed herbs, seeds, rinds, and flowers encased in scented wax that seal the ends of the log or kindling bundles release these scents. **Base notes** form the longest-lasting scent. This will come from the wood, as the other components will burn off quickly.

Here's a method to craft your own scented logs and kindling bundles:

You will need:

A base wood: For fire logs, try to cut your wood with at least one flat surface; this will make it easier to bind dried stalks of herbs and flowers to it. For kindling bundles, you'll want the same kind of wood, cut into 6-to-8-inch length pieces. Each piece should have the girth of a thick twig.

Dried herbs and flowers

Crushed dried herbs, seeds, and flowers

Jute, cotton, hemp, or wool cord in varying colors associated with the season

Wax

Essential oils (if desired, to scent the wax)

Scissors

You'll use the same process to make each seasonal log or bundle; only the unique, individual components will change.

1. For a log, cut five 24-inch lengths of cord. Each one should be long enough to tie around the log and knot it. Cut shorter pieces for the bundles, about 12 inches long.

2. Lay the cords out one after the other, spacing them evenly. The length of the space from the top cord to the bottom one should match the length of the log or pieces of kindling.

3. Center the log or kindling pieces on top of the cords; they'll be the initial means of securing the herbs and flowers to the wood before you bind them with a longer length of cord.

4. Divide the stalks of one of the dried herbs in half. Place one half on the log so that the tips of the flowers line up with the edge of the log, then do the same on the other end. You should have two bundles of flowers on top of the log, flowers facing outward and the cut stems facing each other. For bundles, place the herbs on top of the wood in layers. Don't worry if they fall to the sides, as all the components will be bound together and sealed with the wax.

5. Place the other dried herbs or flowers in the center of the log, on top of what you put down first. If there is a third herb or flower, place it in the center of the log on top of the other two. Adjust the layers so that the entire log is covered and there are no blank spaces.

6. One at a time, tie up each cord to secure the herbs and flowers to the log. Do the same for the kindling bundles.

7. Next, cut a longer length of cord (about 5 feet long for the log, 2–3 feet for the kindling bundles). Lay it out on your workspace, and then place the log or kindling bundle on top of it. Line up the cord with one end of the log or kindling bundle.

8. Carefully pull the cords up so that you have even lengths on both sides, criss-cross them over the herbs and flowers, then wrap them around the back of the log or bundle. Work slowly and methodically, criss-crossing the cords over and under the log until you get to the other end. If you didn't cut a cord long enough to do this, simply knot it off, cut another length of cord, and pick up where you left off. You can bind the log or bundle once or several times.

9. Mix the crushed herbs, flowers, and seeds and place them in a bowl that will accommodate the end of your log or kindling bundle.

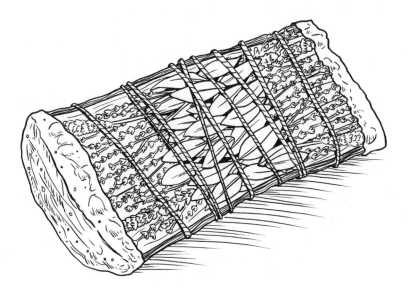

10. Melt the wax and add the essential oil if you're using it.
11. Dip the end of the log into the wax, then quickly into the herb and seed mixture.
12. Repeat step 11 until you have a thick buildup of the mixture and wax on both ends of the log or bundle.

Seasonal Firewood, Flower, and Herb Combinations

The offerings that follow are suggestions. Swap out the different components based on what is available to you or your preferred scents:

Autumn

Autumn scents include the sweetness of straw bundled in bales for hayrides, the earthy damp of trodden leaves, and treats like apple cider and pumpkin pie. Apple wood and dried apples impart a sweet fruitiness, while warm spices dance as top and middle notes for this cozy fire log or kindling bundle.

Wood: Apple
Stalk Herbs and Flowers: Dried apples, cinnamon sticks, golden hay, fallen leaves
Dried and Crushed Herbs, Flowers, and Seeds: Cardamom pods, star anise
Essential Oil: Clove
Cord Colors: Yellow, orange, red, purple

Winter

This winter fire log or kindling bundle delivers the cool sharpness of winter wood, coupled with the cheerful holiday scents of baking gingerbread and clove-studded pomanders.

Wood: Cedar

Stalk Herbs and Flowers: Dried orange slices, rosemary, balsam

Dried and Crushed Herbs, Flowers, and Seeds: Candied orange peel, crystallized ginger, cloves

Essential Oil: Cinnamon

Cord Colors: Red, green, silver

Spring

The essence of spring is freshly cut grass, potent pastel flowers like lilac and hyacinth, and bunnies in the garden. Light birch wood, the princess of the forest, crackles merrily with the new life of this joyful season.

Wood: Birch

Stalk Herbs and Flowers: Lavender, lemon balm, pussywillow branches

Dried and Crushed Herbs, Flowers, and Seeds: Grass clippings, dried lilac flowers, citrus zest

Essential Oil: Bergamot

Cord Colors: Lavender, white, pale green, pale yellow

Summer

Summer's richness is captured in sun-soaked flowers, heady vanilla, and sea spray. Hardwoods like maple and oak have long burn times and release the scent of a traditional summer bonfire.

Wood: Maple, oak

Stalk Herbs and Flowers: Vanilla pods, dried corn husks, yarrow, sunflowers

Dried and Crushed Herbs, Flowers, Seeds: Rosebuds; white,
   black, and pink peppercorns; pink sea salt
Essential Oil: Honeysuckle
Cord Colors: Pink, cerulean, amber, indigo

Resources

These combinations are suggestions. Use the resources below
to discover more aromatic woods for your fireplace or firepit
to warm your heart all year round:

Boeckmann, Catherine. "Best Firewood: Heat Values and Wood-
   Burning Tips." Old Farmer's Almanac. July 3, 2023. https://
   www.almanac.com/content/best-firewood-heat-values-wood
   -burning-tips.

Dume, Raphael. "The Ultimate Guide to the Best Smelling Firewood:
   Unleash Nature's Aromas." *OutdoorDoer* (blog). Last modified July
   14, 2023. https://outdoordoer.com/the-ultimate-guide-to-the
   -best-smelling-firewood-unleash-natures-aromas/.

McDonald, Susan, and Mike Scarpignato. "12 Best Smelling Fire-
   woods (Campfires or Fireplaces)." *RVBlogger*. https://rvblogger
   .com/blog/best-smelling-firewoods-campfires-or-fireplaces/.

Pommells, Kevin. "What Type of Wood Is Best for Bonfires? Full
   Guide." *CamperRules* (blog). https://www.camperrules.com/best
   -wood-for-bonfires#axzz89oQ82c1q.

Indigo Blues

⮞ Rebecca Gilbert ⮜

Around the world, there are at least ten unrelated plant species that contain the precursors of the blue dye we call indigo. What use these compounds provide for the plants is unknown. The methods of extraction and use of the dye differ somewhat from place to place and culture to culture, but they share many similarities because the requirements of the chemical process that form the blue dye are the same. Although this process is complex, it's been figured out by people around the world since ancient times.

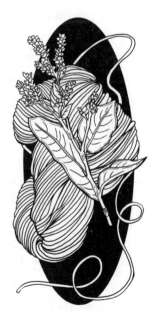

The oldest indigo-dyed material that we know of is from Peru, around 6,200 years old, and knowledge of blue dyes goes back a long way in

Africa, Asia, and Northern Europe as well, although different plants were used to produce them. Since there are lots of plant sources for yellow dyes but very few for green, most antique green fabrics were made with yellow overdyed with an indigo-bearing plant. Robin Hood's traditional Lincoln green, for example, was made with weld (a strong yellow dye) overdyed with woad (the local source for indigo blue).

Three Sources of Dye

Tropical indigo, *Indigofera tinctoria*, grows in hot places, including in the southern United States as far north as the Carolinas. It was so important that the British tried to grow it in their first colony at Jamestown, but without much success. It has a place in American history as the second-largest plantation crop, after tobacco, bringing in one third of the colonies' revenue until the American Revolution. The largest customer for the crop was the British Royal Navy, who bought 80 to 90 percent of the indigo produced and used it to dye navy-blue uniforms. When war was declared, that market suddenly vanished, and the former indigo plantations switched over to growing primarily cotton, while the use of indigo continued on a smaller scale. The knowledge of how to grow, process, and dye with indigo came directly from Africa, and slavers would target areas such as present-day Mali where the people were known to have this valuable knowledge. However, the seeds used to start the indigo plantations came from Peru, where colonial nations had established silver mines. It was to provide labor for those mines that some of the first enslaved Africans were brought to the Americas.

In Europe, tropical indigo eventually replaced the use of woad, the traditional blue dye of ancient Britain and other

Northern European countries. **Woad**, *Isatis tinctoria*, has similar blue precursors, but at a much lower concentration than tropical indigo, which may be as much as ten times stronger. The well-established woad industry in England lobbied successfully to prohibit the use of tropical indigo for almost two hundred years, but eventually the switch was made to the stronger dye plant grown in colonial possessions such as America and Haiti. Woad is now used mainly by traditionalists, reenactors, and historical researchers. It looks somewhat like a narrow-leaved cabbage, with pretty yellow cruciferous flowers. It is not eaten by grazing animals, and is very invasive here in southern New England. It blooms and goes to seed in the second year, so if you are very diligent, you can keep it contained by never letting it flower. However, when I grew it, one fall I missed one bloom and it took me several years to eliminate the seedlings. Luckily, the plants have a distinctive blue-gray color even in the first-year rosette, so I was eventually able to find them all and get rid of them before they reseeded, but I scared myself.

The indigo that I grow and use nowadays is **Japanese indigo**, also called dyer's knotweed, *Persicaria tinctoria*. (If you haven't guessed by now, *tinctoria* is the Latin name for a dye plant.) It's a polygonum native to China and Southeast Asia, in the same family as buckwheat, rhubarb, and dock. It arrived in Japan around the sixth century, where it became a socially important color and gave rise to the fine art form called *shibori*. Although tie-dye is technically related, it doesn't hold the spiritual and cultural meanings that shibori embodies. As with bonsai or flower arranging, the Japanese tradition of shibori requires a philosophical understanding of Japanese culture and aesthetics as well as great technical skill.

Growing Japanese Indigo

Other polygonums include common weeds like smartweed and lady's thumb and their many cousins. However, only *Persicaria tinctoria* has the blue precursors necessary for use as a dye. It's easy to grow here in New England. Wherever you garden, follow schedules and conditions for growing tomatoes. I plant a flat or two indoors in March and then separate the plants and set them out in the garden after the soil has warmed, usually in late May. Japanese indigo transplants easily, growing rootlets from every buried joint. It's the type of plant that will grow roots in a vase if you leave the stems in water. Because of the knotty habit of growth, leafy branches can be broken off throughout the summer and new ones will sprout out of the joints so that multiple harvests can be made in a season. It grows about knee high and has sprays of tiny pink flowers starting around the middle or end of August. It doesn't come back in the garden on its own, either through root or by seed, so it's not invasive.

The only trick to growing it is that the seeds do not keep more than one season. Even sealed in a cool place, very few second-year seeds will grow, and they will be spindly and unthrifty. It's necessary to save seeds from the crop each fall to be planted in the spring. Seed collection is easy—it doesn't cross with its weedy polygonum relatives, so it's just a matter of cutting a bunch of flower heads in the fall. I put them in a paper bag to dry, and store the bag in a closet. Come spring I crumble them up and plant them right out of the bag, spread shallowly in a flat of potting soil, flowers and stems and all, because I'm lazy, and I like to see the pink flower petals on the dark soil. However, it's fine to rub the dried flowers between your hands or through a sieve to collect the tiny seeds, which will be very hard and shiny and range from tan to black in color.

Extracting Pigment

Once you have grown your indigo-bearing plant, the process has only begun. I still have much to learn and my experiments are ongoing, but here's what has worked best for me so far.

A large container (like a tote or barrel) is filled with leaves and stems of freshly picked indigo, and then covered with water. I use hose water, but warm (not hot) water will speed the process. The lid is put on and the contents checked after a day or two. The leaves will turn yellow-brown and the fermenting mess will stink. If you've made compost tea from nettles or comfrey, you'll recognize the smell. The liquid will turn turquoise with a scum of purple-blue floating on top here and there. Some dyers call this stage "mermaid water," while for others it evokes antifreeze. Depending on the temperature, the chemistry of the water, and several other factors, fermentation may take two to seven days. Recognizing when to halt the fermentation process to retain the most pigment is one of the tricks to indigo processing. Sometimes the ideal point is passed in only a couple of hours, especially if the weather is warm. When it seems ready, strain out the leaves. Mermaid water and blue scum are the best indicators. It may take some experimentation to get familiar with the signs. Overfermented indigo will be paler and more greenish. Wear gloves when straining, or your hands will stink for quite a while, even after washing.

The liquid is then aerated by whipping with a whisk made of twigs, pouring from bucket to bucket, or by stirring with a paint mixer. It should start to turn blue after several minutes, especially the foamy bubbles. The next step is to add lime to make the solution alkaline. I use pickling lime (calcium hydroxide), also called slaked lime. It's dissolved in water and added a bit at a time until the solution starts to **flocculate**, or form small clumps of blue pigment that will eventually sink to the bottom. It's allowed to settle until the liquid is tea colored and clear and the blue pigment has formed a sludge on the bottom of the container. This might take a couple of days or more, depending on the size of the particles formed. Now, dip off the liquid as much as possible without disturbing the sludge; this may take several sessions, allowing for resettling in between. Next, pour the sludgy part into a strainer lined with fine cloth such as silk, allow it to drain and dry thoroughly, and then powder the pigment you have refined and collected. A tote full of leaves produces about three tablespoons of indigo powder, which may be stored indefinitely and used to make the dye vat.

Making the Dye Vat

To prepare an indigo vat, three conditions must be met. First, the dyebath must be quite alkaline, about pH 10. Second, oxygen must be removed from the bath. Third, it must be maintained at an evenly warm temperature: between 90 and 100 degrees Fahrenheit (32 and 38°C) for plant fibers like cotton and linen and between 120 and 140 degrees Fahrenheit (49 and 60°C) for animal fibers like silk and wool.

In ancient recipes, the vat is made alkaline with fermented urine or with lye made by dripping water through wood ashes. These days people sometimes use lye, but most modern dyers use ammonia, soda ash, or washing soda, which are safer. All chemicals should be handled with care. Also, consideration should be given to how to safely dispose of the remains of your dye experiments. Alkaline solutions may be neutralized with vinegar before disposal or used to "sweeten" acidic soils.

To remove the oxygen, traditional methods rely on fermentation, and the vat may take weeks to develop. With regular feeding and care of the bacteria, rest periods, and continuous warmth, these vats can last for years. Like with any fermentation process, results are variable. It's also possible to remove oxygen from the vat using chemicals called reducing agents. The one I use is sodium hydrosulphite (sodium dithionite). Other chemical methods use thiox or spectralite (thiourea dioxide) or Rit Color Remover. These chemicals remove the oxygen quickly and effectively but should be treated with respect since they are not naturally as safe or as environmentally friendly as the fermentation methods.

To maintain the required warm temperature for fermentation, much traditional indigo dyeing takes place in hot regions of the world. In Japan, charcoal braziers were used in winter to keep the vats alive. A slow cooker, hot plate, or stove top works for the faster chemical methods, and a light bulb, electric blanket, or heat mat works for longer-running bacterial vats. The solar heat in a summer greenhouse, with nighttime insulation, may be sufficient.

How I Do It

I host a community indigo vat on sunny Sunday afternoons all summer here at the farm. Here is my quick and (relatively) easy and reliable indigo vat recipe.

You will need a large stainless-steel pot containing about 4 gallons of water. The amount of water is not critical, but make sure the pot is large enough to hold the items you wish to dye with plenty of room for movement. Place it on a hot plate or by a fire and warm the pot to a little above body temperature. Add 2 or 3 tablespoons of powdered indigo, homemade or commercially purchased. Add enough soda ash to bring the pH to about 10. The amount will vary with the acidity of the water and other factors, so test with a pH strip. Then add your reducing agent, such as sodium hydrosulphite, a little at a time until the vat looks right. I usually use approximately 20 grams of indigo powder, 200 grams of soda ash, and 200 grams of sodium hydrosulphite.

Once the vat has been made, I keep it going all summer, adding new indigo powder when the dye results start to get lighter, and adding more soda ash now and then if the pH strip indicates that it's not alkaline enough. I need to add more reducing agent each time the vat has sat overnight, because it has absorbed oxygen and turned from green to blue.

Dye Goods
Many plant dyes work better with animal fibers such as wool, silk, alpaca, mohair, and leather. Indigo is equally effective with plant-based fibers like hemp, flax (linen), ramie, and cotton. Indigo also dyes nylon but not polyester. It's terrific for covering up stains or dinginess on a favorite garment and also for decorating gift items such as bandanas, bags, napkins, and pillowcases. Indigo requires no pretreatments (such as mordanting), and items may be washed as they were before. I sometimes give them a final rinse in a mild vinegar solution to make sure the alkalinity of the dyebath has been thoroughly neutralized, but this is not necessary to "set" the color.

Dyeing Goods with the Indigo Vat

Once the vat has been made by dissolving the indigo pigment, bringing the pH to the desired level, removing the oxygen, and gently warming the solution, it is ready to dye. At this point, the vat should be yellow-green below the surface, with a scum of blue and purple on the top where the indigo interacts with the air. It's important not to introduce any more air than necessary into the vat, since it will react with the indigo until the vat no longer works, unless you remove the oxygen again with more reducing agent.

In practice, this means don't stir vigorously or let drips fall and make bubbles, and soak the materials you intend to dye very well. When you squeeze them underwater, they should not release little bubbles but be thoroughly saturated. Wearing gloves, slide the soaked materials into the vat gently, turn them over a few times, wait two to five minutes, and remove. Squeeze the goods while part of them is still touching the solution so the liquid runs off without causing unnecessary bubbles.

When you draw the goods from the vat, they will be yellow-green or grass green. This is the stage at which the indigo will bond with the fibers. Once the dye turns blue, for example in the blue scum on top of the vat, it will not bond with the fibers but will wash off. For successful and permanent dyeing, the bonding must take place in the green stage, and then, once attached, the indigo will pick up extra oxygen from the air or the rinse water, turning from green to blue. This transformation is magical to watch. It usually takes about five minutes to change color completely.

The indigo is now bonded to the fiber. However, a few semiattached bits will wear off with abrasion, which is called **crocking**. If too much indigo has been built up on the fiber at once, crocking can be a problem, with blue coming off on your hands as you knit, for example. Some crocking is normal, as when denim turns lighter blue from wear. Because indigo dye coats and strengthens the material colored with it, it has been traditionally used to dye work clothes everywhere it is found, from the field jackets of rice planters to the blue jeans of cowhands.

To get deep blue shades, it doesn't help to leave the material in the vat longer. Instead, re-dip repeatedly to get darker colors. With the traditional bacterial vat, this can be done up to ten times, resting in between. In some places people would traditionally have their clothing dipped yearly. With the chemical vat, three dips is about the limit, because the chemical will remove some of the color already laid down. But even one dip is enough to transform a dingy or uninteresting garment into something celestial.

Dyeing with indigo is still popular today, partly because the color is so delicious, and perhaps also because it has deep ancestral roots and traditions for the human species. I encourage you to join the conversation with the blue-bearing plants, opening the door to experiment and explore the wide-ranging possibilities of beautiful indigo blues.

Plant
Profiles

Plant Profiles

This section features spotlights on individual herbs, highlighting their cultivation, history, and culinary, crafting, and medicinal uses. Refer to the key below for each plant's sun and water needs, listed in a helpful at-a-glance table.

Key to Plant Needs	
Sun	
Shade	—
Partial shade	☀
Partial sun	☀ ☀
Full sun	☀ ☀ ☀
Water	
Water sparingly	💧
	💧 💧
Water frequently	💧 💧 💧

USDA Hardiness Zones

The United States is organized into zones according to the average lowest annual winter temperature, indicating a threshold for cold tolerance in the area. This USDA Plant Hardiness Zone Map, released in late 2023, uses data collected between 1991 and 2020. For best results, plant herbs that can withstand the climate of their hardiness zone(s) and bring less hardy plants indoors during colder weather. Seek additional resources for high summer temperatures, as these can vary within zones.

It is helpful to keep track of temperatures and frost dates in your neighborhood or check with a local gardening center or university extension for the most up-to-date record. Climate change and local topography will also affect your growing space, so compensate accordingly.

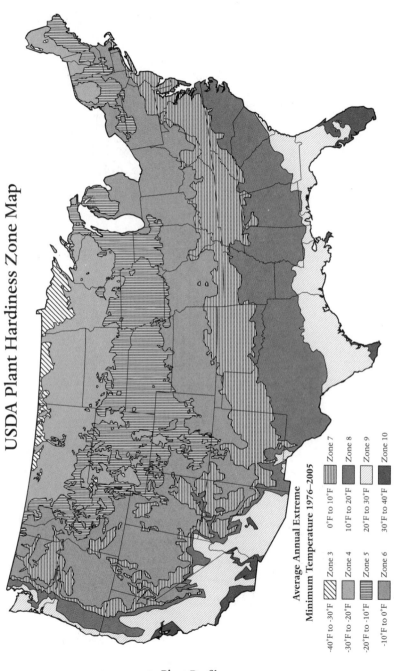

USDA Plant Hardiness Zone Map

Average Annual Extreme
Minimum Temperature 1976–2005

-40°F to -30°F Zone 3   0°F to 10°F Zone 7
-30°F to -20°F Zone 4   10°F to 20°F Zone 8
-20°F to -10°F Zone 5   20°F to 30°F Zone 9
-10°F to 0°F Zone 6   30°F to 40°F Zone 10

USDA Plant Hardiness Zone Map (Cont.)

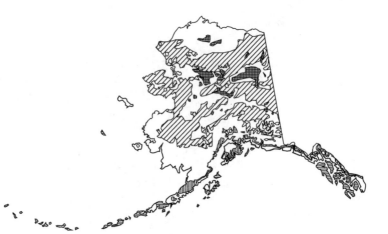

**Average Annual Extreme
Minimum Temperature 1976–2005**

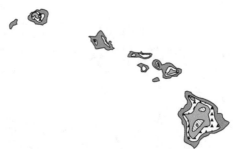

-60°F to -50°F   Zone 1   10°F to 20°F   Zone 8

-50°F to -40°F   Zone 2   20°F to 30°F   Zone 9

-40°F to -30°F   Zone 3   30°F to 40°F   Zone 10

-30°F to -20°F   Zone 4   40°F to 50°F   Zone 11

-20°F to -10°F   Zone 5   50°F to 60°F   Zone 12

-10°F to 0°F   Zone 6

0°F to 10°F   Zone 7

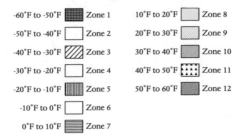

Clove

≫ Anne Sala ≪

As you sit in a trendy coffee shop on a rainy October afternoon, the aroma that surrounds you might hold more than just the scent of the dark roast brewing behind the counter. Could it be . . . *pumpkin spice*? While it may seem this scent has worn out its welcome in our hot drinks, hand soaps, and "limited time only" toaster pastries, practically the whole world has been in love with this smell for centuries. Did your friend order the chai latte? The two scents are not that different.

Both pumpkin spice and chai consist of a combination of spices whose histories have been intertwined since the beginning—and shrouded in mystery. One of the most influential and

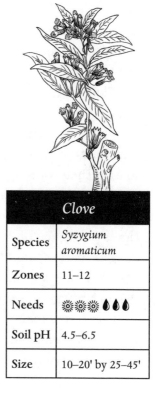

Clove	
Species	*Syzygium aromaticum*
Zones	11–12
Needs	☼☼☼ 💧💧💧
Soil pH	4.5–6.5
Size	10–20' by 25–45'

elusive of these spices was clove. For a long time, only the people who grew cloves knew where they came from, and they alone controlled the distribution throughout the world. As the spice trade expanded, bloody battles were waged as the rest of the world tried to discover the whereabouts of this potent little "nail."

In North America, cloves are familiar to us as a holiday spice—yes, pumpkin pie, but also in apple pie, gingerbread, and mulled cider. They are also used in lots of savory dishes, particularly those made with pork.

Along with the blends mentioned above, cloves are integral to Mexican *mole* sauces, English Worcestershire and HP sauces, French *quatre épices*, Dutch *speculaas* spice mix, Moroccan *ras el hanout*, Tunisian *gâlat dagga*, Ethiopian *berbere*, Arabic *baharat*, Indian *garam masala*, Chinese five-spice powder, and Japanese *tonkatsu* sauce.

Cloves are the dried flower buds of *Syzygium aromaticum*, an evergreen tree in the myrtle family. The spice gets its common name from the Latin word for nail, *clavus*, because the dried buds look like the hobnails the Romans used on the soles of shoes worn by soldiers.

This is the first time I have written an article about a plant that I did not have personal experience growing. Originally, cloves only grew on five volcanic islands in what is now Indonesia (part of the Maluku Islands, or Moluccas): Ternate, Matir, Tidore, Makian, and Bacan. To the rest of the world, this archipelago was known as the Spice Islands.

Clove trees require tropical, partially sunny conditions to thrive, with temperatures remaining above 50 degrees Fahrenheit and ideally within 70 to 85 degrees. The soil must be fertile and moist but not waterlogged. The trees have smooth bark and glossy, oval-shaped green leaves. The leaves have tiny oil glands that release clove oil. The flowers also contain clove oil. Clove trees need to mature about five years before they begin to bloom. Once a clove tree reaches maturity, it can be over twenty-five feet tall and produce up to seventy-five pounds of flower buds per year. Farmers handpick and sort each bud before selling them. The trees can live for hundreds of years but are in their prime at about twenty years old.

Clove oil has a sweet, pungent, woodsy, and almost citrus-like aroma. The spice company McCormick found in their research that high-quality buds can contain 15 to 20 percent clove oil. About 85 percent of that is eugenol, which is also found in basil leaves, cinnamon, and nutmeg (a fellow Spice Island denizen).

Medical Uses

Cloves have been part of Indian culture for thousands of years and are integral to Ayurvedic medicine. Cloves are thought to have a "cooling" effect on the body and can help maintain oral health, reduce phlegm and flatulence, combat fungal infections, and reduce the desire to consume alcohol.

The Chinese also incorporated cloves into their medicine cabinet and used them to support the kidneys, spleen, and stomach. They are considered to be one of the spices that can "warm the interior" and "expel the cold."

Clove is used in holistic medicine as a toothache remedy because eugenol oil has a natural numbing quality. As a young person, I learned the hard way about this particular medicinal power. My friend and I decided to flavor a batch of homemade lip balm with clove oil. It smelled delightful but burned and numbed our lips in a very un-soothing manner!

Clove Incense

In Japan, cloves are used as a traditional incense ingredient. The scent of burning cloves is thought to offer protection and spiritual healing and also to attract wealth.

Powdered cloves can be used as a binder in homemade incense recipes. One can also just light a small pile of clove buds on a ceramic dish or on a charcoal disk specially made to burn loose incense. If you have a campfire or a backyard firepit, add a handful of cloves to the kindling to impart a rich, floral, and resinous scent. Watch out—they crackle and pop!

History

The Maluku Islands were brought to the attention of the "outside world" when Javanese neighbors began trading sago palm for cloves and nutmeg. The Javanese then traded these unique spices with their other trading partners, such as India and China.

When cloves arrived in Europe around the first century CE, the population could not get enough of them. Like many spices that made their way halfway across the world, cloves were very expensive. At first, only royalty and the very rich could afford them. And to show off their wealth, cloves were used to spice everything, from soup, to roast meats, to sweet pastries. One of the reasons cloves were so popular was because a little went a long way. A cook could use just a pinch and it would flavor a large amount of food.

Cloves became integral in the necessary work of food preservation. Not only could the pungent spice mask the flavor of old meat, but it could also help the food last longer because of its antibacterial properties. Cloves, cinnamon, and nutmeg were often combined with stewed meats and brandy, then packed into earthenware crocks and sealed with a layer of fat on top.

As sea travel became more sophisticated, Western countries began to hunt for the source of cloves, which continued to be a closely guarded secret. First, the Portuguese found the Spice Islands in the early 1500s. Later, the English, Spanish, and Dutch found their way there. Battles were waged and early alliances with the ruling classes of the islands fell by the wayside as each foreign country tried to gain complete control of the spice trade.

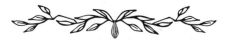

"Somewhere near India is the island containing the Valley of the Cloves. No merchants or sailors have ever been to the valley or have seen the kind of tree that produces cloves: its fruit, they say, is sold by genies."
—Ibrahim ibn Wasif-Shah,
Summary of Marvels, *ca. 1000 CE*

About 100 years later, the Dutch East India Company won out and took severe measures to ensure their hold on the clove market. The Dutch limited the output of spices from the islands to maintain high prices, sometimes setting the excess spices ablaze. They also decided that only clove trees owned by the company could grow, and they burned or cut down all the rest. This was devastating to the native population, especially because they had a long-held tradition of planting a clove tree for every child born, and the life of the tree would foretell the fate of the child.

Unbeknownst to the Dutch, a lone clove tree—now called the Mother Tree or Afo Tree—grew on the side of Mount Gamalama on the island of Ternate. A French diplomat and missionary, Pierre Poivre (Peter Pepper), became aware of the tree's existence in the late 1700s. He managed to smuggle seeds out of the country and brought them to French-occupied territory. They were ultimately planted in Zanzibar, where they thrived. Once these cloves hit the market, it marked the beginning of the end for the Dutch East India Company's long reign.

To this day, the world's demand for cloves continues to be strong. Even so, according to the Observatory of Economic Complexity, clove's home country of Indonesia is high in the charts when it comes to clove consumption. Most of the spice goes into the manufacture of clove-scented cigarettes and not into food, however. Indonesia even has to import cloves from other countries (including the empire-breaking ones from the island of Zanzibar in Tanzania) to support the cigarette market.

A National Food with a Medieval Flavor

Even though the French were pivotal in bringing down the price of spices, they were some of the first to turn up their noses at them. In 2015, I read a fascinating NPR article, "How Snobbery Helped Take the Spice Out of European Cooking." The researchers claimed that once Eastern spices became widely available in Europe, the wealthy no longer wanted to eat heavily spiced food. Instead, "they said things should taste like themselves."

To think France intentionally changed their culinary culture out of what can almost amount to spite seemed particularly cruel to the French colonists who had scattered across Canada and North America in the 1600s. It would not take long before some of their favorite dishes had more in common with medieval food than with the *nouvelle cuisine* beloved by their home country. One example is *tourtière*, a popular colonial dish that is now considered a national food of Canada.

As with a lot of traditional homemade foods, there are as many different ways to cook it as there are cooks, and each family will argue their way is best! Early tourtière recipes called for any manner of filling, from game birds, venison, or other wild game, to pork, beef, and buffalo. Newer recipes often ask for just ground pork or maybe a combination of pork and beef, and sometimes even potatoes. One thing that rarely changes is the addition of spices: cloves, cinnamon, and sometimes allspice and nutmeg. The origin of the name of this dish is also controversial. Is it named after the tourtière pie pan it is made in? Is it named after the type of pigeons, or *tourtes*, that were used as the filling?

While researching tourtière variations, I found recipes that had no spices and instead used herbs, such as sage or savory. It is interesting to think about the events in these families' pasts that led to the absence of spices. Did those first pioneers live too meagerly to afford spices? Or did their ancestors arrive after the culinary rift took place?

⫘ *Tourtière*

I have been making a version of tourtière for many years, but my approach is not beholden to tradition. Without that constraint, the pie becomes very adaptable, especially in terms of the crust. You can top the pie with puff pastry or even a layer of mashed potatoes.

For the recipe below, you are welcome to use your favorite unsweetened pie crust recipe. It is not necessary to have a bottom crust, but having a top and bottom crust is traditional. If you are going to use a skillet or other "unconventional" pan for your pie, you may need more dough than what is produced from a "normal" two-crust recipe. You can make the dough ahead of time (or use store-bought!).

My version contains the controversial addition of mashed potatoes, and I love the heartiness they impart. It is big enough to make two pies. Sometimes I freeze half the recipe for another time, or I bake the whole amount in an iron skillet with high sides. My family enjoys it with a side of HP Sauce—another clove-laced spice mixture!

Here's what you'll need:

For the crust:

> 3 cups unbleached all-purpose flour
>
> 1½ teaspoons salt
>
> 1 cup and 3 tablespoons unsalted butter
>
> ½–¾ cup ice water

For the filling:

> 1–2 tablespoons olive oil
>
> 1½ pounds ground pork
>
> ½ pound ground beef
>
> 1 large onion, minced
>
> 2 garlic cloves, minced
>
> 2 teaspoons salt
>
> ½ teaspoon pepper
>
> ¼–½ teaspoon ground cloves (to taste)

¼–½ teaspoon cinnamon (to taste)

2–3 large potatoes, peeled, boiled and mashed (leftovers from a previous meal are acceptable to use)

½ cup water

Make the Crust

1. Mix the flour and 1½ teaspoons salt in a large bowl. Cut in the butter and rub it into the flour until the butter pieces are about the size of peas.

2. Add the ice water a splash at a time and lightly mix into the flour and butter until it is moistened and begins to form a ball.

3. Gather the dough into 2 balls. Wrap in cling wrap and let it chill in the refrigerator for at least 30 minutes.

4. Before making the filling, roll out the 2 crusts, ensuring they fit the pan you will be using. Return the rolled dough to the refrigerator until needed. It is best to have the crust very cold when you assemble the pie because the filling will be warm.

Make the Filling

1. Preheat the oven to 400°F.

2. Heat olive oil in a large frying pan over medium-high heat. Brown the ground meat and onion until there is very little pink.

3. Push aside the meat mixture to make a space and dump the garlic in the clear spot so it will have a moment to become fragrant before mixing it in with the meat.

4. Assess your pan. Is there an overabundance of grease? If your answer is yes, then spoon out some—but not all—of it.

5. Add salt, pepper, cloves, and cinnamon. Stir to combine.

6. Gently stir in the mashed potatoes. The pan will be very full now, so be careful.

7. Pour in the water, stir to combine, and let it bubble for a few minutes.

8. Assemble the pie in the pie pan or skillet. Make slits in the crust or cut a 1-inch circle in the center. Wrap the edges in foil to prevent burning.

9. Place the pan on a large sheet pan lined with foil or parchment paper to catch drips.

10. Bake for 10 minutes at 400°F. Drop the temperature to 350° and continue baking for about 40 more minutes, until the filling is bubbling.

11. Let cool for at least 10 minutes before serving.

✒ Pumpkin Pie Spice

My recipe box has a pumpkin pie recipe my daughter clipped from the label of an evaporated milk can when she was nine. In her young handwriting, my daughter made some adjustments to the spice components to get the taste "just right." I am sharing her recipe with you so you can recreate that trendy coffeeshop aroma at home. Or use it in your pie. The measurements that follow are enough to season four pies.

You will need:

    4 teaspoons ground cinnamon

    2 teaspoons ginger

    1 teaspoon ground cloves

    ½ teaspoon ground cardamom

Add all ingredients to a bowl and whisk to combine. Store in an airtight container until ready to use.

───

The story of cloves has many high and low points. Despite the greed and sorrow that the spice trade brought, it continues to be an important economic support to the people who first planted the trees in honor of their children. I think it is fitting that this flower bud's heady scent has become a nostalgic connection to the smells of childhood, coming home, and centuries of tradition. I hope the next time you contemplate a pumpkin spice coffee beverage, you order it. Not to be trendy, but to be timeless.

Resources

Betty Crocker's Cookbook. Bridal ed. Hoboken, NJ: Wiley Publishing, 2001.

"Cloves." McCormick Science Institute. Accessed July 20, 2023. https://www.mccormicksscienceinstitute.com/resources/culinary-spices/herbs-spices/cloves.

"Cloves." The Observatory of Economic Complexity. Accessed July 20, 2023. https://oec.world/en/profile/hs/cloves.

Dalby, Andrew. *Dangerous Tastes: The Story of Spices*. Berkeley: University of California Press, 2000. Pages 50–51.

Hancock, James. "The Early History of Clove, Nutmeg & Spice." World History Encyclopedia. October 13, 2021. https://www.worldhistory.org/article/1849/the-early-history-of-clove-nutmeg--mace/.

Knapp Rinella, Heidi. "Sometimes You Just Have to Make It Yourself." *Las Vegas Review-Journal*. May 12, 2015. https://www.reviewjournal.com/entertainment/food/sometimes-you-just-have-to-make-it-yourself/.

Koehler, Jeff. "Spice Migrations: Cloves." *AramcoWorld*. July/August 2021. https://www.aramcoworld.com/Articles/July-2021/Spice-Migrations-Cloves.

Singh, Maanvi. "How Snobbery Helped Take the Spice Out of European Cooking." National Public Radio. March 26, 2015. https://www.npr.org/sections/thesalt/2015/03/26/394339284/how-snobbery-helped-take-the-spice-out-of-european-cooking.

Witty, Helen. *The Good Stuff Cookbook*. New York: Workman Publishing, 1997.

Black Cottonwood

~ Rachael Witt ~

W hen I first met the cottonwood tree, I was told its name
was the "Tacamahac Tree"—the tree
of medicinal resin. Standing 150 feet
below its highest branches, I gazed
up at this tall, powerful, and whimsi-
cal deciduous tree. The leaves were
fluttering in the wind—shiny, dark
green above and silver underneath.
One fell from the branch and slowly
danced its way toward me. It was
shaped like a heart and had toothed
edges. I surveyed the ground and saw
a thick layer of these leaves around
the tree's trunk, blanketing the floor
with nourishment in the form of
mulch. Its gray bark, deeply fur-
rowed, invited my hand to follow
its vertical cervices along its straight

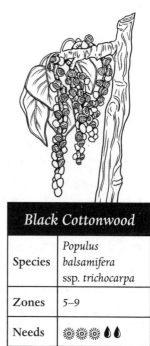

Black Cottonwood	
Species	*Populus balsamifera* ssp. *trichocarpa*
Zones	5–9
Needs	☀☀☀☀ 💧💧
Soil pH	6.0–7.0
Size	20–160' tall

trunk. Apparently, the furrows deepen with age. The tree I met was mature and standing strong among bigleaf maples, alders, and other species of a riparian hedgerow. The tree I met was loved by my mentor and home to many insects, squirrels, and the nest of a bald eagle.

The black cottonwood tree is one of forty species in the genus *Populus*—and the tallest of all. *Populus* is the Latin name for poplar, meaning "tree of the people." It's a member of the willow family (Salicaceae) and, like other trees in this family, cottonwood is a pioneer species that colonizes disturbed and moist sites. The black cottonwood tree grows along the west coast of North America, from Alaska to Baja California, and from the Pacific west coast eastward to the Rocky Mountains. In the mountain west, these trees can adapt to more arid soils, yet they prefer wet areas; hence, these trees are prolific in the Pacific Northwest. To a Washington-based herbalist, black cottonwood is a true ally.

A rooting hormone called **auxin** is found in cottonwood species, helping them propagate from cuttings, wind-borne or waterborne branches, and extended root systems. This tree is known to coppice well and creates new branches and regrowth that can lead to a sustainable supply of wood for biomass (pulp, mulch, shade, etc.). Cottonwood can be a nuisance, and trees are disliked by many for the fact that they are "messy": hard to remove and dropping large branches during wind storms (lending them another name as "widow makers"). People also blame the trees for their seasonal allergies.

The female flowers of cottonwood are called catkins. They are about four inches long and divided into three valves where seeds develop. By early summer, these flowers release their seeds with white fluffy down "cotton" that disperses with the wind. In the Pacific Northwest, this is known as "summer snow." Not all cottonwood trees release this seasonal snow, for *Populus* species are **dioecious**, meaning male flowers and female flowers grow on separate trees, and only the female flowers release cotton-covered seeds.

So why would one be drawn to this tall deciduous tree?

Well, for the *tacamahac*, of course! The medicinal resin found in the leaf buds exudes a fragrance and a golden color that fills the air and catches the eye of an onlooker during a sunny winter's day. For the sake of a forager's well-being, the ability to harvest something so potent during the cold winter days makes for a heart-filled delight.

Harvesting Cottonwood Buds

After the leaves fall and up until the time when the new leaves unfurl in early spring, cottonwood buds are ready to be harvested. In the Pacific Northwest, this can be from early December until late March. I prefer gathering cottonwood buds on a dry, sunny day, as any moisture can create mold or rot the buds and bark.

The best time to harvest is after a windstorm. Downed branches and low-hanging limbs are most likely to be covering the floor underneath a tree stand. These gnarly branches have alternating buds and clusters at the tips. Look for the buds that are pointed and sealed or oozing with red-yellow sap. If the buds are wet and black, they are most likely beginning to decay and should be left to do so.

Remove the buds from the branch and fill a parchment paper bag or a jar that you want to make your medicine in. Since the buds are so sticky, you'll want a harvesting container that can be washed, thrown away, or used specifically for harvesting cottonwood buds. The resin will ruin fabric and stick to paper or plastic.

Some herbalists harvest the twigs with the buds. Due to the medicinal potency of the buds, I tend to focus on the resinous sap medicine. In this case, you will end up with really sticky fingers. To remove the resin from your skin, apply olive oil to cut and lift the resin.

Caution: Those who have allergies to aspirin or bees can be irritated by the resin. This includes contact dermatitis.

To ensure future harvests, it's preferred to harvest downed branches or take a few buds from each tree (leaving the terminal buds). Cuttings or branches can be stuck into the ground to make new roots and future trees in areas you are harvesting.

Storing Cottonwood Buds

Cottonwood buds are best stored in the freezer. Their sap solidifies and their freshness can be preserved for one or two years if the freezer bag is airtight. Buds can be dehydrated as well. However, the dried resin is brittle and less potent, not to mention the resin rarely washes off of drying screens and baskets.

The Medicinal Gifts of Cottonwood Buds

Cottonwood buds are warming and stimulating. I recommend trying a little lick of the fresh sap from the buds. The sap will dry out your mouth and at the same time soothe your throat.

The taste is pungent, astringent, and somewhat bitter. Due to its strong volatile oils, cottonwood buds are antimicrobial and expectorant.

Cottonwood buds are a respiratory ally. As an expectorant, they help expel mucus from the lungs and relieve painful coughs. The buds can be used for wet coughs, lung infections, and inflamed throats. Ethnobotanist Leigh Joseph stated that she learned from a "Squamish knowledge holder, Swanámiya-t Diana Billy, that you can apply the infused oil to your chest as a rub to help with congestion." The bark and buds can also be used as a gargle or throat spray for sore throats and mouth sores.

In the Pacific Northwest, bees use poplar resin to make **propolis** (a.k.a "bee glue"), which seals their hive shut and prevents bacteria, fungus, and disease from entering the colony (if only it deterred the mites . . .). Similarly, humans can use the resin externally as an emollient to protect and soothe our skin. This aromatic antimicrobial helps keep wounds clean while stimulating skin regeneration. Applied externally as a salve or oil, cottonwood buds help accelerate the healing of cuts, scrapes, and burns. I have seen many skin injuries heal with the use of cottonwood oil topically. Some skin symptoms include rashes, irritations, chapped lips, cracked skin, and burns.

My first exposure to cottonwood medicine was in the form of a salve. After coming home from urgent care, bandaged and medicated from chopping off the tip of my pointer finger, I was gifted a tin of homemade cottonwood bud salve. I was told to use Neosporin and keep it wrapped for many months until the tendon and skin started to grow back. The Neosporin did not reduce the pulsing pain in my finger, so I tried the cottonwood salve. It kept the wound clean, it expedited the regrowth of the tissues, and it helped manage the pain. Although my nerves are still tingling many years later, I am grateful for the smooth recovery of my finger with the help of cottonwood.

As a member of the willow family, cottonwood is known to have salicylates in its leaf buds. This helps reduce inflammation associated with pain and further describes the tree's properties as an anti-inflammatory, analgesic, and antirheumatic. It's effective in relieving pain related to swollen joints, carpel tunnel, arthritis, and sore muscles. Topically, an infused oil with the leaf buds can be used on stinging pain associated with burns as well as muscular pains related to menstrual cramping. To best reduce menstrual cramps, I recommend infusing cottonwood buds with castor oil.

External Applications

⚘ Cottonwood Oil

This is a topical oil that can be applied to sprains, strains, and pains. It can also be applied to cuts or skin irritations. For stronger or more specific actions, combine with other herbal oils. I love to make a "trauma oil" with equal parts oils of cottonwood, mugwort, St. John's wort, and arnica. For a "cell renewal blend," combine oils of cottonwood, calendula, and comfrey.

You will need:

> 1 part fresh cottonwood buds
>
> 2 parts olive oil (or carrier oil of choice)

Let the buds sit on parchment paper overnight to allow any moisture to dissipate.

Place the buds into a large jar and cover them with oil. Cover the jar with cheesecloth and place it in a warm location away from moisture (windowsills, on top of the refrigerator, near a heat vent, etc.).

Stir the buds and oil at least once a day for the first week. After 2 weeks, remove the cheesecloth and cover with a solid lid. Place the jar in a warm setting to infuse the buds slowly in the oil for at least 2 more weeks.

I have infused cottonwood buds from 6 months to 1 year and find that the oil is more potent. The antibacterial properties of the bud help preserve the oil as long as no moisture is introduced. The oil will turn as dark as the buds' sap and have a strong aroma to go with.

Strain the buds from the oil. Pour the infused oil in an amber glass jar. Keep it in a dark, cool place.

This oil will last at least 1 year or until its aroma begins to fade.

☙ *Wonderful First Aid Salve*

This salve is one of my best-selling remedies. It reduces swelling; prevents infection; soothes dry, cracked, irritated skin; and promotes skin cell regeneration. It can be used on open wounds and is pet friendly!

You will need:

2 ounces (28 grams) beeswax

1 cup cottonwood oil

½ cup plantain leaf oil

½ cup yarrow oil

Melt the beeswax in a double boiler or saucepan on low heat.

Once the beeswax has melted, add the herbal infused oils. This most likely will solidify part of the beeswax again. Stir well to melt and combine the wax and oil.

As the oil and wax melt into liquid again, pour the combination into salve tins or glass jars.

Let the salve cool and harden. Cover with a lid, label, and store in a cool place. Cottonwood-based salves can last 2 or more years.

Internal Uses

ᐧ Throat Elixir

Whether it is used for a sore throat or taken as a digestif, this elixir is delicious! I like to take it by the spoonful or add it to a hot toddy when I am sick.

You will need:

   1 cup fresh black cottonwood buds

   2 cups brandy

   ½ cup honey

Harvest fresh cottonwood buds into a jar.

Pour the brandy and honey over the buds.

Cover with lid and shake thoroughly until the honey is dissolved.

Label the jar and let it sit for at least 4 weeks in a cold, dark place. Flip the jar every week to further disperse the honey into the brandy.

Strain out the buds and pour the elixir into an amber glass jar. Store it in a dark, cool, dry place.

Take 1 teaspoon of elixir by mouth or combine it with a tea to soothe a sore throat. This can be taken 3 to 5 times per day depending on the severity of the symptoms.

This elixir can be poured into a 2-ounce spray bottle and used as a throat spray. Make sure the honey is fully dissolved to prevent clogging the sprayer. Spray onto the back of the throat 3 to 12 times a day as needed.

The Magical Gifts of Cottonwood Trees

Black cottonwood offers more medicine than just that of its resin. If the leaves don't speak to your heart, then perhaps the tall stature and maturity of the tree will. This tree is a witness to many stories and can hold the pains, woes, and burdens of many people. Its physical presence can bring balance and strength among turbulent waters. Black cottonwood teaches how to stay grounded and wail in great storms. May you find support and renewal with your local cottonwood trees.

Resources

Apelian, Nicole, and Claude Davis. *The Lost Book of Herbal Remedies*. Claude Davis, 2019.

"Black Cottonwood (*Populus trichocarpa*)." Oregon Wood Innovation Center. Oregon State University. Accessed July 30, 2023. https://owic.oregonstate.edu/black-cottonwood-populus-trichocarpa.

De la Forêt, Rosalee, and Emily Han. *Wild Remedies: How to Forage Healing Foods and Craft Your Own Herbal Medicine*. Carlsbad, CA: Hay House, 2020.

Gray, Beverley. *The Boreal Herbal: Wild Food and Medicine Plants of the North*. Whitehorse, Yukon: Aroma Borealis Press, 2011.

Hammerquist, Natalie. *A Visual Guide to Medicinal Plants of the Pacific Northwest*. Self-published, 2022.

Joseph, Leigh. *Held by the Land*. New York: Wellfleet, 2023. Pages 80–81.

Kloos, Scott. *Pacific Northwest Medicinal Plants: Identify, Harvest, and Use 120 Wild Herbs for Health and Wellness.* Portland, OR: Timber Press, 2017.

Moore, Michael. *Medicinal Plants of the Pacific West.* Santa Fe: Museum of New Mexico Press, 1993.

"Populus balsamifera L. ssp. *trichocarpa* (Torr. & A. Gray ex Hook.) Brayshaw." PLANTS Database. United States Department of Agriculture. Accessed July 30, 2023. https://plants.usda.gov/home/plantProfile?symbol=POBAT.

Peonies

⤞ Charlie Rainbow Wolf ⤝

*P*eonies. The very sound of the word conjures up familiar memories of my mother's garden. She was passionate about flowers and had different kinds of peony bushes all around the house. In my youth, I thought they were called "penny" bushes, and I loved that, as Penny was the name of my childhood best friend. When I moved to England, they were featured in many of the cottage gardens in the village. I cannot think about peonies without feeling a bit nostalgic.

Peonies never seem to have gone out of fashion, either. Yes, there are those who think they are outdated, who rip them out and plant whatever happens to be en vogue at the time,

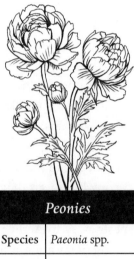

Peonies	
Species	*Paeonia* spp.
Zones	3–8
Needs	☀☀☀ 💧💧
Soil pH	6.0–7.0
Size	2–3' wide & tall

but they always seem to endure somehow. There are now thousands of varieties, with new ones being developed all the time.

Background

Peonies are ancient. They have been cultivated for well over 4,000 years—possibly longer—originating in Asia and then spreading around the world. Today, peonies are considered native in Asia, Europe, and North America. It's the state flower for Indiana.

Peonies are perennial herbaceous plants that die down after the frost and return the following spring. We always say that spring really is on its way when we see the peonies poking through the mulch! Peonies require very little attention, and when properly cared for, they're said to live for up to 100 years! They're fairly disease resistant, but plant them where you think they're going to stay, as they don't really like to be moved once established. They like full sun, and they don't like strong winds or heavy rains.

One of the biggest complaints I've heard about peonies is *ants*. It's true that ants like the sweet, sticky substance on the peony buds, but they won't hurt the plant. In fact, I've heard experienced folks say that the ants keep other, more harmful pests away from the plants.

Peonies are not just eye candy, though. They are also edible and medicinal. In herbal medicine, the peony (*Paeonia lactiflora*) is used to boost the immune system and brighten the mood. In the context of herbal medicine, "white peony" and "red peony" refer to the peeled or unpeeled root, rather than the color of the flowers.

Growing Peonies

Here in the United States, peonies grow in most regions. They are considered hardy perennials in zones 3 to 8. They perform best where there are cold winters and may struggle a bit in zone 8 and hotter.

Peonies love the sun and like to have at least six hours of sunlight per day. Ours are near the crab apple trees and get shaded during the heat of the afternoon, but they still perform well. The general rule of thumb is the more sun they get, the better they'll bloom.

Plant peonies in loose fertile soil that is well drained. We always add some compost when we plant new peonies, as well as some all-purpose fertilizer. Bare-root peonies can be planted in spring or autumn; they don't mind the frost. If you're planting something grown in a pot from a nursery, I've always found it best to plant in spring after the danger of frost has passed.

Dig a hole about 12 inches wide and 12 inches deep. Loosen the soil well and add compost and fertilizer. Add the removed soil and mix well, then remove enough of the mix to leave a hole approximately 15 inches deep. Position the peony root so the growing tips are just under the soil line, no more than ¾ inch—if planted too deeply, they'll produce foliage but no flowers. Cover the root and water when needed. Remember, they don't like wet feet—in fact, they're quite drought tolerant once they're adapted. It will take them 2 or 3 years to settle in, but once they're established, they will develop a big root system and grow into a prolific plant that will last for years.

Peonies make great additions to perennial gardens, being one of the first to flower in spring. Here in Illinois, we usually see the flowers around Memorial Day, starting with the paler pink ones and finishing with the darker fuchsia ones. I remember seeing peonies used as low hedging in England, often in alternating colors.

Peonies will thrive as a low shrub as long as they are in well-drained soil and their air and sunlight requirements are met. They don't like to be cramped or crowded. Their flowers are often top heavy, so consider putting a peony cage around them as they start to grow in the spring. All peonies flower, but some flower earlier than others. Different cultivars extend the flowering season.

Peonies are rarely bothered by diseases, but we have had some minor issues with a *Botrytis* fungus, which makes spots on the leaves. This happens when we've had a warm, wet spring. It's not killed the plant, and it has been easily treated by removing the damaged area and thinning out the peonies in the autumn.

Caring for peonies is easy. After the flowers have faded, remove them with sharp scissors to stop them from going to seed. This enables that energy to go back into the foliage, ultimately preparing the plant for next year's blooms. After the first frost, when the foliage has yellowed, cut it back to about seven centimeters above the surface of the soil. Add a bit of fertilizer the following spring when the shoots are six inches tall, and the peonies will pretty much take care of themselves!

Moving or dividing peonies is best done in the fall when they're starting to sleep, rather than in the spring when they're starting to grow. Cut the foliage short and dig a hole big enough for the entire root ball, which can be *big*! Be careful not to break off smaller roots—I've moved the same peony three times because a bit of the root had been left behind in its original spot! Divide a peony when it is lifted by cutting off a section of the root or using a spade to cut pieces away from the mother plant. Replant immediately and water well.

More Than Just a Pretty Face

I love peonies and will always have them in my yarden (yard + garden = yarden). They aren't just pretty; they are useful! We eat them. I make jelly and cordial with the peony petals, and my husband makes peony wine.

All the recipes start in the same manner. I gather the flowers as they've just reached fully open, early in the morning when the dew is gone but before the sun gets too hot. I have a bucket of cold water nearby, and I plunge the flower heads in that to remove any ants that might be hitching a ride. Then I bring the flowers into the house.

The petals have to be removed from their bases. If this is too easy, the flowers are too far open, and if it is not easy, then the flowers are not open quite enough. It does not matter what color flowers you choose, as they all produce the same-tasting results, but the darker red peonies do seem to leave a bit more color when it comes to jelly—or that may just be my imagination!

⫸ Peony Jelly

This jelly recipe uses a simple ratio: I use roughly 1 cup of packed peony petals per 1 cup of water to make jelly. To make four 8-ounce jars of jelly, you'll need 4 cups of petals and 4 cups of water and an equal measure of sugar—4 cups in this instance.

You will need:

- 4 cups peony petals
- 4 cups of water
- 4 cups of sugar
- 2 tablespoons lemon juice
- 1 box pectin (1.75 ounces)

Sterile canning jars and their 2-piece ring lids, a large pan of boiling water for the hot water bath, and a ladle are also needed—and I use the canning "grabbers" (which look like large tongs) for handling the hot jars.

Make a tea from the peony petals by putting them in a heatproof dish and pouring the required measurement of boiling water over them. They will begin to release their color almost immediately. Cover them and let them steep overnight.

Strain out the petals and pour the peony tea into a sauce-pan, adding more water if necessary to bring the liquid back up to a measurement of 4 cups. Bring this to a boil, then add the lemon juice and the pectin. Bring the mix back to a rolling boil for a minute or two before adding the sugar. *Do not add the sugar before or at the same time as the pectin or your jelly won't set.* I learned the hard way; you can learn from my mistakes!

I sterilize my jelly jars while waiting for the tea to boil. There are many ways of doing this. I like the idea of using the dishwasher to clean and sterilize them until they're needed, but I don't have a dishwasher! Therefore, I put them in a clean sink and pour boiling water to cover them, adding a bit of my husband's sanitizer that he uses for his home brew equipment.

Jars can also be sterilized in an oven by washing and rins-ing them carefully, then placing them on a rack in an oven at 320°F (160°C). This temperature is important; lower than this, the jars might not sterilize properly, and higher than this, they might break. Keep them in the oven for 15 minutes, then remove them using canning grabbers.

Another method of sterilization is to boil the jars in the canning bath water; simply add the jars, rings, and lids to the water and bring it to a boil for 10–15 minutes. Follow the instructions for your area, because elevation will make a difference. Use the canning grabbers to remove the jars and lids from the boiling water and be careful to avoid burns.

Test the jelly for readiness. It won't take long for the sugar to dissolve, and it is ready to go into the bottles when a drop of jelly solidifies on a cold plate (I keep one in the fridge for this purpose). It will still look very runny at this stage but that's okay. Skim off any foam from the pectin and ladle the jelly into the sterile jelly jars, immediately covering them with the sterile lids and rings.

Tighten the rings and then lower the filled jars into the canning bath of boiling water. *Be careful*—both the water and the jars will be very hot! It's possible to buy racks that go into the bottom of the canning bath to separate the jars, but I don't bother with one; I use a silicone mat in the bottom and it suffices. The water must cover the lids of the jars by at least a half inch to seal them properly. Process the jelly in the canning bath for 10–16 minutes, again, depending on altitude. A general rule of thumb is to increase the time in the canning bath by 5 minutes per every 3,000 feet above sea level. Remove the jars from the water bath with the canning grabbers, then carefully dry them and give the rings a final tighten before setting them aside to cool.

I use the mason jar lids that have the button in the middle. It will *thwop* and become depressed when the seal takes as the jar has cooled. Sometimes a jar won't *thwop*. It's still okay to eat the jelly: simply treat it like an open jar and keep it in the fridge, using it within 6 weeks and discarding it should it start to look or smell funky as time passes.

Use the peony jelly in the same way that you would any store-bought jelly. I put it between layers on summer sandwich cakes, spread it on crackers with cream cheese, and have it on toast with tea as a snack. Mine always comes out a jewel-like pale rose color no matter what color the peony blossoms were. It's sweet with a slightly acidic aftertaste, and when I eat the jelly in the cold winter months, I'm reminded that the peonies are only sleeping and that spring is right around the corner.

⚶ *Peony Cordial*

This is made in the same way as peony jelly, but omit the pectin. Dissolve the sugar in the peony tea (with the added lemon), bring to a boil until the sugar has dissolved, and then place into the sterilized canning jars and process in the same way. The cordial is lovely over ice as a cool drink. Use 1 part cordial to 4 parts water, or more if a stronger taste is desired. It also makes a wonderful addition to gimlets and other summer beverages. Yields 4 cups.

⚶ *Peony Wine*

Brewing is really my husband's domain, but one year I nagged him to try peony wine, and it promised to be so good that we made it again the next year! Peony wine is a sweet wine that is pale pink in color, and I think it is absolutely gorgeous. It's a bit more complicated than making jelly, but well worth the effort!

Starred ingredients and materials in the following lists are available from home brew shops, online retailers, and sometimes local pharmacies.

For the wine:

6 cups peony petals

2 quarts purified or filtered water, plus another 2 quarts

6 cups sugar

4 cups white grape juice

4 tablespoons lemon juice, or the juice of 2 lemons

1 teaspoon yeast nutrient*

⅛ teaspoon wine tannin (or half a cup of strong black tea)

1 camden tablet, crushed*

1 packet of wine yeast (look for alcohol tolerance under 16%)*

1 teaspoon potassium sorbate*

Winemaking equipment:

2-gallon fermenting bucket with lid

Home brew sanitizer*

2 glass carboys, sometimes called demijohns

Plastic tubing to siphon the liquid from one container to another

Rubber bung and an airlock, sometimes called a water-lock

Bottles. We use flip-top beer bottles ("Grolsch" bottles), but it's a matter of personal choice. Some say wine keeps better in the long-necked corked and sealed wine bottles, but it never lasts long enough in our home to make a difference.

Corks and a corker if you're using that kind of bottle

We start our flower wines in the fermenting bucket because it's easier to strain the **must** (unfermented liquid) off the sediment this way. The petals go in the bottom of the bucket first. The water and the sugar are heated on the stove until the sugar is dissolved; once they are cool, this sugar water is poured over the flower petals. Cool this overnight, then add the grape juice (optional), lemon juice, yeast nutrient, and camden tablet. Leave the must in a cool, dark place for another 24 hours, then add the yeast. Return the bucket of must to a cool, dark place for 5–7 days (we usually wait a week). Now it's time to take the liquid off the petals.

Sterilize the carboy and the plastic tubing with sanitizer. Add another 2 quarts of purified water to the petals in the bucket. Stir, then strain the liquid off the petals into the carboy. This is done by elevating the bucket higher than the carboy, and using the tubing to siphon the liquid off the petals.

Once the liquid is in the carboy, sterilize the air lock and attach it to the rubber bung. Place the bung in the neck of the carboy, and put the carboy back into a cool, dark place for at least another week. If there is sediment on the bottom of the carboy after a week, the wine will need to be siphoned into the second (sterilized) carboy. This process is called **racking**, and it is necessary to keep removing the young wine off any sediment, because deposits on the bottom of the fermenting liquid can give the wine an unpleasant taste.

Keep checking the wine every 4 weeks, and rack again should sediment build up. As the wine ferments, it will clear, and bottom deposits will be slow to form. Once the wine is clear and there has been no sediment for several weeks, it is time to bottle!

Add 1 teaspoon potassium sorbate to the carboy to ensure that all fermentation has ceased (no stirring or shaking is necessary), and then siphon the wine into sterilized bottles.

It's still not ready to drink, though, and this is the agonizing part! It has to age at least 6 months. We try to leave ours 1 year, but it rarely makes it longer than 9 months!

Resources

Here are a few titles I recommend for further reading on growing peonies, making preserves, and winemaking:

Making Homemade Wine. Storey's Country Wisdom Bulletin A-75. North Adams, MA: Storey Publishing, 1981.

Massaccesi, Raymond. *Winemaker's Recipe Handbook*. Self-published, 1976.

US Department of Agriculture. *Complete Guide to Home Canning and Preserving*. 2nd rev. ed. Mineola, NY: Dover Publications, 1999.

Vargas, Pattie, and Rich Gulling. *Making Wild Wines & Meads: 125 Unusual Recipes Using Herbs, Fruits, Flowers & More*. North Adams, MA: Storey Publishing, 1999.

Weber, Stephanie J. *How Not to Kill a Peony: An Owner's Manual*. Self-published, 2018.

Strawberry

～ Lupa ～

Summertime brings a wide variety of fresh fruit, and perhaps none is so iconic as the strawberry. This luscious red fruit is a sweet addition to cakes and other treats, a colorful garnish in salad, and enjoyable by itself too. And it's easy to grow!

There over two dozen species and hybrids in the genus *Fragaria*. The Northern Hemisphere features the bulk of wild species, from *Fragaria nipponica*, which is only found on the Japanese islands of Honshu and Yakushima, to *Fragaria cascadensis*, which was discovered in 2012 to be a unique species in the Cascade Mountains of Oregon. They all tend to have three serrated green leaves on a single stem, and female plants produce

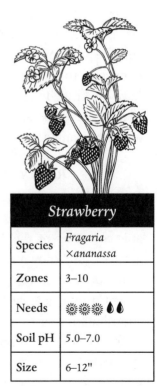

Strawberry	
Species	*Fragaria* ×*ananassa*
Zones	3–10
Needs	☀☀☀ 💧💧
Soil pH	5.0–7.0
Size	6–12"

flowers with five white petals that mature into red fruits. These fruits are generally much smaller than those found at the grocery store or farmers' market.

The fruit is not a true berry; instead, the red flesh of the strawberry is known as a **receptacle**, and the tiny "seeds" are actually dry fruits called **achenes**. Inside each achene is one seed, which will grow if planted. This is somewhat similar to the situation with rose hips; if you cut one open, you will find many little achenes that are often mistaken for the seeds themselves. Dandelions, maples, and other familiar plants also have achenes that encapsulate their true seeds.

While strawberries may certainly reproduce through seeds, they reproduce even more quickly with runners. These slender stems reach out from the parent plant, and once they find a suitable patch of earth, they take root. The plants may remain connected to each other for a while even after the newer ones have established themselves. A plant produced from a runner that has developed sufficiently mature roots can be detached and transplanted.

Domesticating the Strawberry

Our modern domesticated strawberry is a hybrid known as *Fragaria* ×*ananassa*, but its parents have roots on both oceanic coastlines of the Americas. The wild strawberry (*F. virginiana*), also known as the Virginia strawberry, grows across much of the United States and Canada, though it is largely absent from dry areas like grasslands and deserts. The other contributing species, the beach strawberry (*F. chiloensis*), can be found along the Pacific coastline of North America, from southern Alaska to extreme southern California, and then in Ecuador and southern Chile in South America.

Originally it was *F. vesca*, the woodland strawberry, that was cultivated in Europe as far back as the Roman era. *F. ×ananassa* was an accidental discovery; French botanists in the mid-1700s found that when they planted beach strawberries near wild strawberries, the beach strawberries produced much larger fruits than normal, notes botanist Arther C. Gibson. This led to further research into the existence of both female and male strawberry plants and how this complicated hybridization.

Until recently, strawberry cultivation was primarily done in private farms and gardens. In the early twentieth century, the United States government began allocating money for widespread strawberry cultivation, creating a new cash crop. This sped up selective breeding for plants whose fruit would be larger and more capable of handling long journeys by train, truck, or airplane. Within a few decades, the domesticated strawberry developed in the United States was being cultivated elsewhere, even displacing the woodland strawberry's popularity in Europe.

Breeding strawberries could be a challenge, particularly when experimenting with crossbreeding different species. Not all members of the genus *Fragaria* have the same number of chromosomes, and often species with different numbers of chromosomes cannot reproduce, or if they do, the offspring is sterile. Some strawberry species are diploid, meaning they have two pairs of chromosomes. Others are tetraploid (four pairs) or octoploid (eight pairs), and even hexadecaploid species with sixteen pairs of chromosomes are known.

Today, most strawberries are cultivated the old-fashioned way. Pollinators such as bees carry pollen from one flower to another, facilitating fertilization. Runners also allow strawberry plants to reproduce quickly in ideal conditions. In recent years, genetic engineering has allowed specific traits to be introduced. For example, a gene from the Arctic flounder (*Liopsetta glacialis*) that confers cold resistance was transferred to strawberry plants. As a result, these plants were better able to survive cold temperatures that would otherwise have killed them. (They did not, of course, display any other traits of the flounder, such as a fishy flavor.)

Cultivating Strawberries

You don't need to be a genetic engineer to be able to grow some strawberries for yourself, though. While not absolutely foolproof, strawberries are one of the easier plants to cultivate, even if you don't have a lot of space.

What you do need is a dedicated sunny spot. The more sunlight the plants get throughout the day, the more they'll produce. Six hours of direct sunlight is the absolute minimum. Avoid planting strawberries near large trees and shrubs that may compete with them for water, unless you're able to provide plenty of extra hydration.

Because strawberry roots are relatively short, they don't need incredibly deep soil, though they certainly appreciate depth. However, you'll want to make sure your plants have plenty of room to spread out as they create runners. If you choose to plant them directly in the ground, you'll need to be mindful of weeds and other competitors that may shade out these low-growing plants.

Pay attention to your soil too. Clay-heavy soil may be too thick for your strawberries, and poorly draining soil can cause the roots to rot. Sandy or loamy soil is a better option, and the plants will be much happier if you add a lot of compost and other organic amendments. Mulching around individual plants will curb weeds, but will also make it tougher for runners to take root.

It's also possible to grow strawberries in containers with good drainage. A standard pot will work, especially if it is wide enough to allow room for runners. There are even special hanging containers for growing strawberries, though these can be quickly overgrown. A hard plastic wading pool full of potting soil is a great option if you have room, as it is deep enough for the plants' roots but allows plenty of space for runners. Any good potting soil will work, but, again, you may wish to amend with compost or other organic material.

Strawberries can be challenging to grow from seed, so you're better off getting some starts. Most of what's available in North America will be cultivars of *F. ×ananassa*, but heirloom seed and start companies sometimes have old or rare cultivars of *F. vesca* (often labeled "alpine" strawberries.)

Strawberry starts can be planted even if the risk of frost hasn't yet passed. The important thing is to make sure you choose a cultivar that is adapted to your hardiness zone. United States zones 7 through 10 can plant as early as December, but zones 3 to 4 should wait until early May. Your strawberries will need regular watering, as they like damp soil. Those in containers will need to be watered more frequently in hot weather, as the soil dries out faster.

When will you get fruit? Well, that depends on the variety you planted. **June-bearing strawberries** generally produce fruit once in early summer, while **ever-bearing strawberries** may fruit all summer. However, some experts recommend that for the first year your strawberries should not be allowed to grow fruit at all, so that they put all their energy into becoming stronger and healthier overall and producing more and better fruit in the next seasons. If you choose to go this route, you'll need to remove all flowers and runners for the first year, and then allow them to produce fruit the following year.

Protecting Your Plants and Berries

In warmer climates, strawberries should have no trouble dealing with winter cold. However, once the temperatures drop into the twenties or below, it's best to cover them with a few inches of straw or mulch. They can handle a light frost or two, and this can help harden them off. Harder frosts, though, can cause serious damage.

There's nothing worse than walking out to pick your fresh, new strawberries—only to find something else got to them first! Birds are a common culprit here, and who can blame them for wanting a nice, sweet meal? To protect your strawberries, build a wooden framework over their container or bed, and drape a mesh fabric over it; make sure the holes in the mesh aren't too small, or else this will essentially be a shade cloth. This structure will still allow sunlight and water in, but keep the birds out.

Insects and other invertebrates can be trickier, though not all of them are harmful. Cutworms, thrips, and tarnished plant bugs can all do serious damage to strawberry plants; fruit flies are an additional nuisance. Slugs and snails will eat the fruit. Removing weeds takes away shelter these small animals need, and refraining from using pesticides and other chemicals invites beneficial insects that can help keep pests under control, as can planting a variety of native plants in your garden.

Cooking with Strawberries

Let's say you are successful in growing your strawberries. Of course, you're welcome to pick them straight off the plant and eat the sun-warmed fruit right then and there. But you have plenty of other options too.

Fresh strawberries are an amazing addition to all sorts of salads. Fruit salad is a classic, but a green salad will benefit from the sweet red pop of sliced strawberries. A poppyseed or balsamic dressing adds a nice tang that goes well with the fruity flavor. And try adding in pecans or pumpkin seeds for a complementary crunch.

Strawberries also go well with many cheeses. Mashed strawberries or a homemade strawberry jam blends well with cream or neufchâtel cheese and makes a fabulous spread on bread, crackers, bagels, and more. Goat cheese also pairs well with strawberries, the strong flavor of the cheese being balanced out by the berries' sweetness. Try stuffing the strawberries with cheese; a little chocolate sauce adds a surprising dimension.

If you are an omnivore, you can try making a sauce with strawberries and balsamic vinegar to serve over beef or pork. Break out the grill, and barbecue chicken pieces in a sweet barbecue sauce, then garnish with fresh strawberries. In a hurry? Use strawberry jam as a base for a meat sauce, adding in whatever other flavors you want to include.

But it's dessert where the strawberry truly shines. From strawberry cheesecake to strawberry ice cream, along with pies, cobblers, and even cookies, there's no end to the possibilities. I want to share one of my favorite recipes: simple strawberry tarts.

➳ Simple Strawberry Tarts

    1 whole pie crust, either store-bought or homemade

    ½ tablespoon cornstarch

    ¼ cup water

    3 cups sliced fresh strawberries

    ½ cup sugar (white, brown, or raw)

Grease the cups in a 12-muffin tin, then line each one with a thin layer of pie crust. Bake at 350°F for 15–20 minutes or until golden brown, and set these tart crusts aside to cool. Make a slurry of the cornstarch and water. Pour the slurry, strawberries, and sugar into a saucepan. Bring to a boil while stirring frequently, then lower the heat to a simmer and continue to stir until the mixture thickens. Remove from heat, allow to cool for 5–10 minutes, then spoon the mixture into the tart crusts. If desired, top with whipped cream or vanilla ice cream, then serve.

Strawberry Allergy

If you have never eaten strawberries before, a little caution is advised. A small number of people are allergic to this plant, including the berries. It especially crops up in those who have pollen allergies, as the allergen is not the strawberry itself but tree or other pollen on its textured surface. This can cause significant reactions, such as oral swelling and itching and, if swallowed, significant gastrointestinal symptoms, among others. In rare cases, anaphylaxis and other severe symptoms may result. Washing, peeling, or cooking strawberries does not seem to ease the allergy.

However, an allergy to the strawberry itself may also be at fault. A particular anthocyanin—one of the natural pigments that gives the fruit its red color—has an associated protein that can cause allergic reactions, note Swedish researchers for Innovations Report. Interestingly enough, strawberry cultivars that produce a white or otherwise pale fruit, such as the pineberry, may not produce the same allergic reaction.

Resources

"The Chemistry of Strawberry Allergy." Innovations Report. June 21, 2005. https://www.innovations-report.com/health-and-medicine/report-45626/.

Darrow, G. M. *The Strawberry: History, Breeding, and Physiology*. New York: Holt, Rinehart, and Winston, 1966.

Erik. "Growing Strawberries." Strawberry Plants. April 19, 2018. https://strawberryplants.org/growing-strawberries.

Giampieri, Francesca, Sara Tulipani, Josè M. Alvarez-Suarez, Josè L. Quiles, Bruno Mezzetti, and Maurizio Battino. "The Strawberry: Composition, Nutritional Quality, and Impact on Human Health." *Nutrition* 28, no. 1 (January 2012): 9–19. https://doi.org/10.1016/j.nut.2011.08.009.

Gibson, Arthur C. "Strawberry, the Maiden with Runners." Economic Botany. Accessed September 13, 2023. Wayback Machine archive. https://web.archive.org/web/20100706193324/http://www.botgard.ucla.edu/html/botanytextbooks/economicbotany/Fragaria/index.html.

Munger, Gregory T. "Fragaria vesca." Fire Effects Information System. United States Department of Agriculture. 2006. https://www.fs.usda.gov/database/feis/plants/forb/fraves/all.html.

Gardening
Resources

Companion Planting Guide

Group together plants that complement each other by deterring certain pests, absorbing different amounts of nutrients from the soil, shading their neighbors, and enhancing friends' flavors. This table of herbs and common garden vegetables offers suggestions for plants to pair together and plants to keep separated.

Plant	Good Pairing	Poor Pairing
Anise	Coriander	Carrot, basil, rue
Asparagus	Tomato, parsley, basil, lovage, Asteraceae spp.	
Basil	Tomato, peppers, oregano, asparagus	Rue, sage, anise
Beans	Tomato, carrot, cucumber, cabbage, corn, cauliflower, potato	Gladiola, fennel, *Allium* spp.
Bee balm	Tomato, echinacea, yarrow, catnip	
Beet	Onions, cabbage, lettuce, mint, catnip, kohlrabi, lovage	Pole bean, field mustard
Bell pepper	Tomato, eggplant, coriander, basil	Kohlrabi
Borage	Tomato, squash, strawberry	
Broccoli	Aromatics, beans, celery, potato, onion, oregano, pennyroyal, dill, sage, beet	Tomato, pole bean, strawberry, peppers
Cabbage	Mint, sage, thyme, tomato, chamomile, hyssop, pennyroyal, dill, rosemary, sage	Strawberry, grape, tomato
Carrot	Peas, lettuce, chive, radish, leek, onion, sage, rosemary, tomato	Dill, anise, chamomile

Plant	Good Pairing	Poor Pairing
Catnip	Bee balm, cucumber, chamomile, mint	
Celery	Leek, tomato, bush bean, cabbage, cauliflower, carrot, garlic	Lovage
Chamomile	Peppermint, beans, peas, onion, cabbage, cucumber, catnip, dill, tomato, pumpkin, squash	
Chervil	Radish, lettuce, broccoli	
Chive	Carrot, *Brassica* spp., tomato, parsley	Bush bean, potato, peas, soybean
Coriander/cilantro	*Plant anywhere*	Fennel
Corn	Potato, beans, peas, melon, squash, pumpkin, sunflower, soybean, cucumber	Quack grass, wheat, straw, tomato
Cucumber	Beans, cabbage, radish, sunflower, lettuce, broccoli, squash, corn, peas, leek, nasturtium, onion	Aromatic herbs, sage, potato, rue
Dill	Cabbage, lettuce, onion, cucumber	Carrot, caraway, tomato
Echinacea	Bee balm	
Eggplant	Catnip, green beans, lettuce, kale, redroot pigweed	
Fennel	*Isolate; disliked by all garden plants*	
Garlic	Tomato, rose	Beans, peas
Hyssop	*Most plants*	Radish
Kohlrabi	Green bean, onion, beet, cucumber	Tomato, strawberry, pole bean
Lavender	*Plant anywhere*	
Leek	Onion, celery, carrot, celeriac	Bush bean, soy bean, pole bean, pea

Plant	Good Pairing	Poor Pairing
Lemon balm	*All vegetables*, particularly squash, pumpkin	
Lettuce	Strawberry, cucumber, carrot, radish, dill	Pole bean, tomato
Lovage	*Most plants*, especially cucumber, beans, beet, *Brassica* spp., onion, leek, potato, tomato	Celery
Marjoram	*Plant anywhere*	
Melon	Corn, peas, morning glory	Potato, gourd
Mint	Cabbage, tomato, nettle	Parsley, rue
Nasturtium	Cabbage, cucumber, potato, pumpkin, radish	
Onion	Beets, chamomile, carrot, lettuce, strawberry, tomato, kohlrabi, summer savory	Peas, beans, sage
Oregano	*Most plants*	
Parsley	Tomato, asparagus, carrot, onion, rose	Mint, *Allium* spp.
Parsnip	Peas	
Peas	Radish, carrot, corn, cucumbers, bean, tomato, spinach, turnip, aromatic herbs	*Allium* spp., gladiola
Potato	Beans, corn, peas, cabbage, eggplant, catnip, horseradish, watermelon, nasturtium, flax	Pumpkin, raspberry, sunflower, tomato, orach, black walnut, cucumber, squash
Pumpkin	Corn, lemon balm	Potato
Radish	Peas, lettuce, nasturtium, chervil, cucumber	Hyssop
Rose	Rue, tomato, garlic, parsley, tansy	*Any plant within 1 ft. radius*
Rosemary	Rue, sage	

Plant	Good Pairing	Poor Pairing
Sage	Rosemary	Rue, onion
Spinach	Strawberry, garlic	
Squash	Nasturtium, corn, mint, catnip, radish, borage, lemon balm	Potato
Strawberry	Borage, bush bean, spinach, rue, lettuce	*Brassica* spp., garlic, kohlrabi
Tarragon	*Plant anywhere*	
Thyme	*Plant anywhere*	
Tomato	Asparagus, parsley, chive, onion, carrot, marigold, nasturtium, bee balm, nettle, garlic, celery, borage	Black walnut, dill, fennel, potato, *Brassica* spp., corn
Turnip	Peas, beans, brussels sprout, leek	Potato, tomato
Yarrow	*Plant anywhere*, especially with medicinal herbs	

For more information on companion planting, you may wish to consult the following resources:

Mayer, Dale. *The Complete Guide to Companion Planting: Everything You Need to Know to Make Your Garden Successful*. Ocala, FL: Atlantic Publishing, 2010.

Philbrick, Helen. *Companion Plants and How to Use Them*. Edinburgh, UK: Floris Books, 2016.

Riotte, Louise. *Carrots Love Tomatoes: Secrets of Companion Planting for Successful Gardening*. Pownal, VT: Storey Books, 1988.

Cooking with Herbs and Spices

Elevate your cooking with herbs and spices. Remember, a little goes a long way!

Herb	Flavor Pairings	Health Benefits
Anise	Salads, slaws, roasted vegetables	Reduces nausea, gas, and bloating. May relieve infant colic. May help menstrual pain. Loosens sputum in respiratory illnesses.
Basil	Pesto and other pasta sauces, salads	Eases stomach cramps, nausea, indigestion, and colic. Mild sedative action.
Borage	Soups	Soothes respiratory congestion. Eases sore, inflamed skin. Mild diuretic properties.
Cayenne	Adds a spicy heat to soups, sauces, and main courses	Stimulates blood flow. Relieves joint and muscle pain. Treats gas and diarrhea.
Chamomile	Desserts, teas	Used for nausea, indigestion, gas pains, bloating, and colic. Relaxes tense muscles. Eases menstrual cramps. Promotes relaxation and sleep.
Chervil	Soups, salads, and sauces	Settles and supports digestion. Mild diuretic properties. Useful in treating minor skin irritations.
Chive	Salads, potato dishes, sauces	Rich in antioxidants. May benefit insomnia. Contributes to strong bones.
Coriander/ cilantro	Soups, picante sauces, salsas	Treats mild digestive disorders. Counters nervous tensions. Sweetens breath.

Herb	Flavor Pairings	Health Benefits
Dill	Cold salads and fish dishes	Treats all types of digestive disorders, including colic. Sweetens breath. Mild diuretic.
Echinacea	Teas	Supports immune function. May treat or prevent infection.
Fennel	Salads, stir-fry, vegetable dishes	Settles stomach pain, relieves bloating, and stimulates appetite. May help treat kidney stones and bladder infections. Mild expectorant. Eye wash treats conjunctivitis.
Garlic	All types of meat and vegetable dishes as well as soup stocks and bone broths	Antiseptic: aids in wound healing. Treats and may prevent infections. Benefits the heart and circulatory system.
Ginger	Chicken, pork, stir-fry, gingerbread and ginger cookies	Treats all types of digestive disorders. Stimulates circulation. Soothes colds and flu.
Hyssop	Chicken, pasta sauces, light soups	Useful in treating respiratory problems and bronchitis. Expectorant. Soothes the digestive tract.
Jasmine	Chicken dishes, fruit desserts	Relieves tension and provides mild sedation. May be helpful in depression. Soothes dry or sensitive skin.
Lavender	Chicken, fruit dishes, ice cream	Soothes and calms the nerves. Relieves indigestion, gas, and colic. May relax airways in asthma.

Herb	Flavor Pairings	Health Benefits
Lemon balm	Soups, sauces, seafood dishes	Soothes and calms the nerves. Treats mild anxiety and depression. Helps heal wounds.
Lemongrass	Marinades, stir-fries, curries, spice rubs	Treats all types of digestive disorders. Reduces fever. May reduce pain.
Lemon verbena	Beverages, any recipe asking for lemon zest	Calms digestive problems and treats stomach pain. Gently sedative.
Lovage	Soups, lovage pesto, lentils	Acts as a digestive and respiratory tonic. Has diuretic and antimicrobial actions. Boosts circulation. Helps menstrual pain.
Marigold	Soups, salads, rice dishes	Effective treatment of minor wounds, insect bites, sunburn, acne, and other skin irritations. Benefits menstrual pain and excessive bleeding.
Marjoram	Vegetables, soups, tomato dishes, sausages	Calms the digestive system. Stimulates appetite.
Nasturtium	Nasturtium pesto, salad dressings, salads	Strong antibiotic properties. Treats wounds and respiratory infections.
Oregano	Chicken, tomato sauces and dishes	Strong antiseptic properties. Stimulates bile production. Eases flatulence.
Parsley	Soups, stocks, bone broths	Highly nutritious. Strong diuretic action and may help treat cystitis. Benefits gout, rheumatism, and arthritis.
Peppermint	Desserts, teas	Treats all types of digestive disorders. May help headaches.

Herb	Flavor Pairings	Health Benefits
Purslane	Salads	Treats digestive and bladder ailments. Mild antibiotic effects.
Rosemary	Roasted red meats, potato dishes, grilled foods	Stimulates circulation. May stimulate the adrenal glands. Elevates mood and may benefit depression.
Sage	Chicken, duck, and pork	Relieves pain in sore throats. May help treat menstrual and menopausal disorders.
Spinach	Sautéed, soups, salads, spinach pesto, stuffed in chicken, ravioli	Iron-rich; supports healthy blood and iron stores.
Summer savory	Mushrooms, vegetables, quiche	Treats digestive and respiratory issues.
Tarragon	Chicken, fish, vegetables, sauces—"classic French cooking"	Stimulates digestion. Promotes sleep—mildly sedative. Induces menstruation.
Thyme	Soups, stews, tomato-based sauces	May treat infections. Soothes sore throats and hay fever. Can help expel parasites. Relieves minor skin irritations.
Winter-green	Ice cream, candies, desserts	Strong anti-inflammatory and antiseptic properties. Treats arthritis and rheumatism. Relieves flatulence.
Winter savory	Beans, meats, vegetables	Treats digestive and respiratory issues. Antibacterial properties.
Yarrow	Salad dressings, infused oils	Helps heal minor wounds. Eases menstrual pain and heavy flow. Tonic properties.

Gardening Techniques

Gardeners are creative people who are always on the lookout for the most efficient, interesting, and beautiful ways to grow their favorite plants. Whether you need to save money, reduce your workload, or keep plants indoors, the following gardening techniques are just a sampling of the many ways to grow your very own bountiful garden.

Barrel

Lidless plastic food-grade barrels or drums are set on raised supports. Before the barrel is filled with soil, slits are cut into the sides of the barrel and shaped into pockets. A PVC pipe is perforated with holes and set into the center and out of the bottom of the barrel as a delivery tool for watering, draining, fertilizing, and feeding the optional worm farm.

Strengths

Initial cost is moderate. Retains moisture, warms quickly, drains well, takes up little space, maximizes growing area, and repels burrowing rodents. Little weeding or back-bending required.

Weaknesses

Not always attractive, initially labor intensive, requires special tools to modify. Not generally suited for crops that are deep-rooted, large vining, or traditionally grown in rows, such as corn.

Hügelkultur

These permanent raised beds utilize decomposing logs and woody brush that have been stacked into a pyramidal form on top of the soil's surface or in shallow trenches and then packed and covered with eight to ten inches of soil, compost, and well-rotted manure. The rotting wood encourages soil biota while holding and releasing moisture to plants, much like a sponge. English pronunciation: "hoogle-culture."

Strengths
Vertical form warms quickly, drains well, reduces watering needs, increases overall planting surface, and reduces bending chores. In time the rotting wood breaks down into humus-rich soil.

Weaknesses
Labor-intensive construction and mulch tends to slide down sides. Requires two to three years of nitrogen supplementation, repeated soaking, and filling sunken voids with soil. Voids can also be attractive to rodents and snakes in the first few years.

Hydroponic
Hydroponics is based on a closed (greenhouse) system relying on carefully timed circulation of nutrient-enriched water flowing through a soilless growing medium in which plants grow. Aerial parts are supported above the water by rafts and, at times, vertical supports. With the addition of fish tanks to the system, hydroponics becomes aquaponics.

Strengths
Customizable to any size. Versatile, efficient, productive, and weedless. Produce stays clean.

Weaknesses
Large systems are expensive and complicated to set up and maintain; require multiple inputs of heat, light, and nutrients; and are limited to certain crop types.

Lasagna
Based on sheet composting, lasagna gardens are built up in layers, starting with paper or cardboard that is placed on top of turf-covered or tilled ground to smother weeds and feed ground worm activity. This is then covered in repeating layers of peat moss, compost, leaves, wood chips, manure, and yard waste (green, brown, green), which eventually break down into rich, humusy soil.

Strengths
Excellent natural method to enrich poor soils, utilizes organic waste, supports soil biota, and improves drainage while reducing the need for fertilizers and excessive watering.

Weaknesses
Initially labor intensive and the proper breakdown of bed materials takes months, so is not suited to "quick" gardening. Requires ready and abundant sources of clean, unsprayed, organic materials.

Ruth Stout
This "no work" garden is based on deep, permanent layers of progressively rotting straw mulch, which simultaneously builds soil, feeds plants, blocks weeds, and reduces watering. Seeds and plants are placed into the lower decomposed layers. Fresh straw is added as plants grow and kept at a depth of eight or more inches.

Strengths

No tilling, few weeds, reduced watering and fertilizing. Warms quickly in the spring and prevents winter heaving. An excellent method for rocky, sandy, or clay soils.

Weaknesses

Requires an abundance of straw each season, which can be expensive and difficult to transport, move, and store. Deep mulch may encourage burrowing rodents and provide shelter for slugs, insect pests, and diseases.

Soil Bag

This simple method utilizes one or more twenty- to forty-pound bags of commercial potting soil or topsoil simply laid out flat on turf, mulch, or wood pallets. A rectangular hole is cut into the top and drainage holes are punched through the bottom. A light dusting of fertilizer is mixed in and plants and seeds are sown.

Strengths

Super easy, weed-free, no-till garden and a great way to start an in-ground garden. Fun for kids and those without a yard.

Weaknesses

Limited to shallow-rooted crops, needs consistent watering and fertilizing, and may flood in heavy rains. Cats may find this an attractive litter box.

Straw Bale

One or more square, string-bound straw bales are placed cut side up either directly on the ground or on top of a weed barrier and soaked with water for several days or even months and treated with nitrogen to help speed the decomposition of the straw. Alternatively, bales can be overwintered in place before using. Once ready, bales are parted down the center, filled with soil and compost, and planted with seeds or starts.

Strengths

Good on poor soils, even concrete. No tilling required, few weeds, handicap accessible, versatile, easy to configure, and renter-friendly. Spent bales make excellent mulch.

Weaknesses

Straw bales can be expensive, heavy, and difficult to transport. These gardens can initially be labor intensive, require frequent watering and fertilizing, and must be replaced every one or two seasons. Nitrogen from treated bales can leach into the local environment and affect the watershed.

Square Foot

This modern take on French Intensive gardening utilizes raised beds filled with a special soilless blend enclosed in a box frame that is further divided into twelve-by-twelve-inch squares, or one square foot. Each square is planted or seeded based on the correct spacing requirements of each plant. Large crops, like tomatoes, are planted one to a square, while small crops like radishes are planted sixteen to a square.

Strengths

Proper plant spacing utilizes space, increases yields, and reduces weeds. Adding trellises increases growing capacity. Raised beds drain well, warm quickly, hold mulch, look tidy, and are easy to mow around.

Weaknesses

Initial construction is expensive, labor intensive, and often impermanent. Requires frequent watering in dry spells, and not all crops are suitable. Grids can be tedious to use and do not remove the gardener's need to learn proper plant spacing.

Vertical

Vertical gardens make use of nontraditional gardening space in two ways. The first is by training vining and climbing plants onto trellises, arbors, or fences and growing in raised beds, pots, urns, or tubs. The second is by firmly securing containers, troughs, rain gutters, or vertical garden felt pockets onto permanent frames supported by fences, walls, or other sturdy vertical structures. These gardens are typically irrigated by automatic drip or hydroponic systems. Soilless options are available.

Strengths

Attractive and weed-free indoor-outdoor garden perfect for small yards, renters, and disabled persons. Helps hide ugly structures and views and defines outdoor spaces.

Weaknesses

Construction of large systems and very sturdy structures can be initially expensive or labor intensive. Not conducive to all garden crops and requires frequent and consistent applications of moisture and fertilizer.

2025 Themed Garden Plans

The Soothing Garden

While the act of gardening alone is a therapy for the soul, there are many plants with natural properties that calm the nerves and boost mood. These herbs are easily grown in a home garden bed and can be used fresh or dried to brew into infusions. Drink them as tea or pour them into the bath for a relaxing soak to calm frazzled nerves, elevate outlook, and allow you to regain your enjoyment of life.

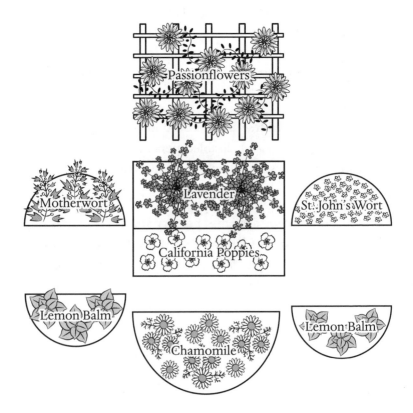

The Mediterranean Herb Garden

For a garden of fragrant and easy-to-grow culinary herbs that will even flourish in patio pots, try going Mediterranean, as in the two options below. Mediterranean herbs are not just practical, but they are also attractive garden plants loved by bees and butterflies, and as they are herbs of antiquity, each has a history filled with legends and lore. Learning about a plant's history deepens the experience of learning how to grow and use it. Mediterranean herbs are sun-loving herbs and need to be planted in a spot with full sun exposure and well-draining soil.

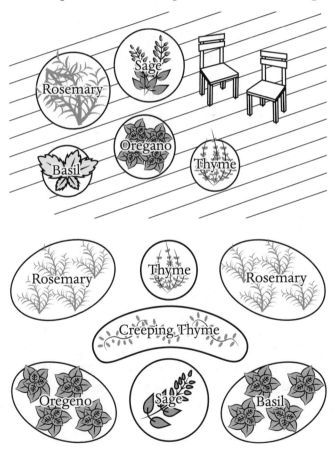

Salsa Garden

One of the best pieces of advice I have for a beginner gardener is "grow what you love." That goes double for the vegetable garden. Tomatoes may be the most popular plant in vegetable plots across the country, but you don't need to include them in your garden plan if you hate eating them. Use the space you have to grow your favorites.

Me? I love tomatoes. Give me a plate of heirloom tomato slices drizzled with olive oil, a caprese sandwich, or a slice of tomato frittata, and I'm happy. For me, the flavor of summer would not be complete without a plethora of tomatoes. Growing up in the Southwest gave me a love for fresh salsa. In the summer, I heap salsa on breakfast eggs, use it to dress my salad greens, and mash it into ripe avocados for a quick guacamole. Having an abundance of salsa ingredients available right outside my door makes putting together a fresh batch quick and convenient.

Enjoy two layouts of this garden on the following page.

Garden Fresh Salsa

    3 cups chopped tomatoes
    1 cup diced onion
    ¼ cup fresh cilantro leaves, stems removed
    3 tablespoons lime juice
    2 hot peppers (serrano or jalapeño), finely chopped
    3 cloves of garlic, minced
    Salt and pepper to taste

Stir together ingredients in a medium bowl. Serve chunky for a pico de gallo, or blend it in a food processor for a salsa fresca.

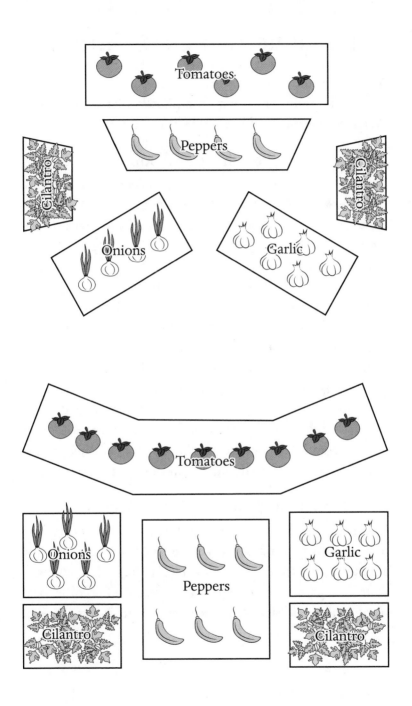

Planning Your 2025 Garden

Prepare your soil by loosening and fertilizing. Use the grid on the right, enlarging on a photocopier if needed, to sketch your growing space and identify sunny and shady areas.

Plot Shade and Sun

For new beds, watch your yard or growing space for a day, checking at regular intervals (such as once an hour), and note the areas that receive sun and shade. These will shift over the course of your growing season. Plant accordingly.

Diagram Your Space

Consider each plant's spacing needs before planting. Vining plants, such as cucumbers, will sprawl out and require trellising or a greater growing area than root crops like carrots. Be sure to avoid pairing plants that naturally compete or harm each other (see the Companion Planting Guide on page 262).

Also consider if your annual plants need to be rotated. Some herbs will reseed, some can be planted in the same place year after year, and some may need to be moved after depleting the soil of certain nutrients during the previous growing season.

Determine Your Last Spring Frost Date

Using data from previous years, estimate the last spring frost date for your area and note what you'll need to plant before or after this date. Refer to seed packets, plant tags, and experts at your local garden center or university extension for the ideal planting time for each plant. Keep track of frost dates here:

| 2022 | 2023 | 2024 | 2025 |

Growing Space Grid

☐ = _____ inches/feet

January

Task	Date

Notes:

_____

_____

_____

_____

_____

_____

_____

JANUARY

			1	2	3	4
5	◑	7	8	9	10	11
12	○	14	15	16	17	18
19	20	◐	22	23	24	25
26	27	28	●	30	31	

Beer Slug Trap

Slug, hold my beer. If someone doesn't finish their beverage, don't toss it. Place shallow bowls throughout your garden and fill them with leftover beer. Slugs will go for that before they go for your plants and will drown themselves— along with your garden sorrows.

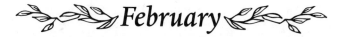

February

Task	Date

Notes:

_____

_____

_____

_____

_____

_____

_____

_____

Black Tea Fertilizer

Fertilize your plants with a cuppa. Loose-leaf black tea can double up as a fertilizer. Green tea will impart its antioxidant benefits to you. Its leaves will give your plant's soil a shot of iron.

FEBRUARY

						1
2	3	4	◑	6	7	8
9	10	11	○	13	14	15
16	17	18	19	◐	21	22
23	24	25	26	●	28	

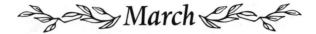

March

Task	Date

Notes:

_____

_____

_____

_____

_____

_____

_____

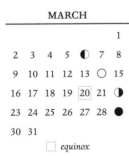

MARCH

						1
2	3	4	5	◐ 7		8
9	10	11	12	13	○	15
16	17	18	19	20	21	◑
23	24	25	26	27	28	●
30	31					

equinox

Prevent Fungi with Chamomile

Chamomile tea (used sparingly) helps protect seedlings while they're germinating. Give your plants an occasional spritz of cooled chamomile tea to keep fungi at bay.

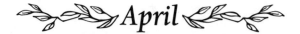

April

Task	Date

Notes:

_____

_____

_____

_____

_____

_____

_____

There's Nothing Coffee Can't Fix

Coffee grounds—high in copper, magnesium, nitrogen, phosphorus, and potassium—will give a boost to your soil. Plus, coffee is antifungal, anti-slug, and anti-snail. Straight-up black coffee diluted with water will add acidity to your soil. Use sparingly, once a month at most.

APRIL

		1	2	3	◐	5
6	7	8	9	10	11	○
13	14	15	16	17	18	19
◑	21	22	23	24	25	26
●	28	29	30			

May

Task	Date

Notes:

_____

_____

_____

_____

_____

_____

_____

_____

MAY

				1	2	3
◐	5	6	7	8	9	10
11	○	13	14	15	16	17
18	19	◑	21	22	23	24
25	●	27	28	29	30	31

Got Milk?

Milk's vitamin B and calcium are good for plants too, especially tomatoes. Don't pour milk directly onto your plants, as too much can be harmful. Dilute with water and spray sparingly.

June

Task	Date

Notes:

_____

_____

_____

_____

_____

_____

_____

Antibacterial Lemonade

Lemonade, that cool summer refresher, can also give a boost to your plants. Add a couple of tablespoons in your full watering can to help kill bacteria.

JUNE

1	◐	3	4	5	6	7
8	9	10	○	12	13	14
15	16	17	◑	19	20	21
22	23	24	●	26	27	28
29	30					

⬚ solstice

July

Task	Date

Notes:

_____

_____

_____

_____

_____

_____

_____

JULY				
	1 ◐	3	4	5
6	7 8 9 ○	11	12	
13	14 15 16 ◑	18	19	
20	21 22 23 ●	25	26	
27	28 29 30 31			

Orange Juice Fertilizer

A little OJ mixed with water will act as a fertilizer for your plants. Like all human beverages, use sparingly (a couple of tablespoons every now and then). Too much will over-acidify the soil and be harmful to your plants.

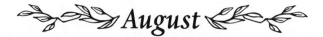

August

Task	Date

Notes:

_____

_____

_____

_____

_____

_____

_____

Seltzer Boost

Try giving your plants a little seltzer (not cold from the fridge) for growth and greener leaves. Sparkling mineral water may also add extra nutrients to your plants' soil.

AUGUST

					◑	2
3	4	5	6	7	8	○
10	11	12	13	14	15	◐
17	18	19	20	21	22	●
24	25	26	27	28	29	30
◑						

September

Task	Date

Notes:

_____

_____

_____

_____

_____

_____

_____

SEPTEMBER

		1	2	3	4	5	6
○		8	9	10	11	12	13
◑		15	16	17	18	19	20
●		22	23	24	25	26	27
28	◐	30					

equinox

Cola in Your Compost

*Add some flat cola to your compost pile.
The shot of sugar will provide a natural boost
to the decaying process. It can also be used
to kill weeds.*

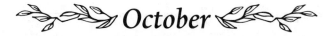

October

Task	Date

Notes:

_____

_____

_____

_____

_____

_____

_____

_____

Vodka Pesticide and Fungicide

Vodka can be used as a pesticide and fungicide. Mix 1 quart water with about ⅛ cup vodka and ⅛ cup dish liquid. Swirl together and spritz your plants to keep bugs at bay.

OCTOBER

				1	2	3	4
5	○	7	8	9	10	11
12	◐	14	15	16	17	18
19	20	●	22	23	24	25
26	27	28	◑	30	31	

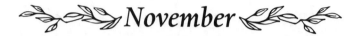# November

Task	Date

Notes:

_____

_____

_____

_____

_____

_____

_____

NOVEMBER

						1
2	3	4	○	6	7	8
9	10	11	◑	13	14	15
16	17	18	19	●	21	22
23	24	25	26	27	◐	29
30						

Cut-Flower Refresher

Add a little wine and 1 teaspoon sugar to 4 cups water and spray on cut flowers to help them last longer. Wine can also accelerate the composting process. Mix a couple of teaspoons of wine with water (at least 4 cups) to fertilize your houseplants.

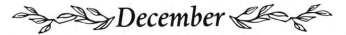

December

Task	Date

Notes:

_____

_____

_____

_____

_____

_____

_____

_____

Recycled Cloches

Save your clear drink bottles—plastic and glass! Cut off the neck and you have a handmade cloche that can create humidity for plants and seedlings.

DECEMBER

	1	2	3	○	5	6
7	8	9	10	◑	12	13
14	15	16	17	18	●	20
21	22	23	24	25	26	◐
28	29	30	31			

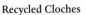 solstice

Gardening by the Moon

It is believed that the moon's gravitational pull extends beyond Earth's oceans, affecting the moisture in the soil, seeds, and plants. Some gardeners utilize this timing to strategically plan various gardening activities. Here's how:

Gardening by Moon Phase

During the waxing moon (from new moon to full moon), plant annuals, crops that need to be seeded anew each year, and those that produce their yield above the ground. During the waning moon (from full moon to new moon), plant biennials, perennials, and bulb and root plants. As a rule, these are plants that produce below the ground.

These are not hard-and-fast divisions. If you can't plant during the first quarter, plant during the second, and vice versa. There are many plants that seem to do equally well planted in either quarter, such as watermelon, hay, and cereals and grains.

First Quarter (Waxing): The first quarter begins with the new moon. Plant annuals that produce their yield above the ground and are generally of the leafy kind that produce their seed outside their fruit. Examples are asparagus, broccoli, brussels sprouts, cabbage, cauliflower, celery, cress, endive, kohlrabi, lettuce, parsley, and spinach. Cucumbers are an exception, as they do best in the first quarter rather than the second, even though the seeds are inside the fruit. Also in the first quarter, plant cereals and grains.

Second Quarter (Waxing): Plant annuals that produce their yield above ground and are generally the viney types that produce their seed inside the fruit. Examples include beans, eggplant, melons, peas, peppers, pumpkins, squash, and tomatoes.

Third Quarter (Waning): The third quarter begins with the full moon. Plant biennials, perennials, and bulb and root plants. Also plant trees, shrubs, berries, beets, carrots, onions, parsnips, peanuts, potatoes, radishes, rhubarb, rutabagas, strawberries, turnips, winter wheat, and grapes.

Fourth Quarter (Waning): This is the best time to cultivate, turn sod, pull weeds, and destroy pests of all kinds, especially when the moon is in the barren signs of Aries, Leo, Virgo, Gemini, Aquarius, and Sagittarius.

Gardening by Moon Sign

Some gardeners include the influence of the twelve astrological signs in their lunar gardening as well. The moon changes sign roughly every two and a half days.

Moon in Aries: Barren and dry. Used for destroying noxious growth, weeds, pests, and so on, and for cultivating.

Moon in Taurus: Productive and moist. Used for planting many crops, particularly potatoes and root crops, and when hardiness is important. Also used for lettuce, cabbage, and similar leafy vegetables.

Moon in Gemini: Barren and dry. Used for destroying noxious growths, weeds, and pests, and for cultivation.

Moon in Cancer: Very fruitful and moist. This is the most productive sign, used extensively for planting and irrigation.

Moon in Leo: Barren and dry. This is the most barren sign, used only for killing weeds and for cultivation.

Moon in Virgo: Barren and moist. Good for cultivation and destroying weeds and pests.

Moon in Libra: Semi-fruitful and moist. Used for planting many crops and producing good pulp growth and roots. A very good sign for flowers and vines. Also used for seeding hay, corn fodder, etc.

Moon in Scorpio: Very fruitful and moist. Nearly as productive as Cancer; used for the same purposes. Especially good for vine growth and sturdiness.

Moon in Sagittarius: Barren and dry. Used for planting onions, for seeding hay, and for cultivation.

Moon in Capricorn: Productive and dry. Used for planting potatoes, tubers, etc.

Moon in Aquarius: Barren and dry. Used for cultivation and destroying noxious growths, weeds, and pests.

Moon in Pisces: Very fruitful and moist. Used along with Cancer and Scorpio, and especially good for root growth.

Planting Guide for Moon Phase and Sign

The following table shows how to combine the moon's quarters and signs to choose the best planting dates for crops, flowers, and trees.

Plant	Quarter	Sign
Annuals	1st or 2nd	*See specific entry*
Apple trees	2nd or 3rd	Cancer, Pisces, Taurus
Asparagus	1st	Cancer, Scorpio, Pisces
Barley	1st or 2nd	Cancer, Pisces, Libra, Capricorn
Beans	2nd	Cancer, Pisces, Libra, Taurus
Beets	3rd	Cancer, Pisces, Libra, Capricorn
Berries	2nd	Cancer, Scorpio, Pisces
Biennials	3rd or 4th	*See specific entry*
Broccoli	1st	Cancer, Scorpio, Pisces, Libra
Brussels sprouts	1st	Cancer, Scorpio, Pisces, Libra

Plant	Quarter	Sign
Buckwheat	1st or 2nd	Capricorn
Bulbs	3rd	Cancer, Scorpio, Pisces
Bulbs for seed	2nd or 3rd	*See specific entry*
Cabbage	1st	Cancer, Scorpio, Pisces, Taurus
Cantaloupes	1st or 2nd	Cancer, Scorpio, Pisces, Taurus
Carrots	3rd	Cancer, Scorpio, Pisces, Libra
Cauliflower	1st	Cancer, Scorpio, Pisces, Libra
Celery	1st	Cancer, Scorpio, Pisces
Cereals	1st or 2nd	Cancer, Scorpio, Pisces, Libra
Chard	1st or 2nd	Cancer, Scorpio, Pisces
Chicory	2nd or 3rd	Cancer, Scorpio, Pisces
Clover	1st or 2nd	Cancer, Scorpio, Pisces
Corn	1st	Cancer, Scorpio, Pisces
Corn for fodder	1st or 2nd	Libra
Cress	1st	Cancer, Scorpio, Pisces
Cucumbers	1st	Cancer, Scorpio, Pisces
Deciduous trees	2nd or 3rd	Cancer, Scorpio, Pisces, Virgo
Eggplant	2nd	Cancer, Scorpio, Pisces, Libra
Endive	1st	Cancer, Scorpio, Pisces, Libra
Flowers	1st	Taurus, Virgo, Cancer, Scorpio, Pisces, Libra
Garlic	3rd	Libra, Taurus, Pisces
Gourds	1st or 2nd	Cancer, Scorpio, Pisces, Libra
Melons	2nd	Cancer, Scorpio, Pisces
Onion seeds	2nd	Scorpio, Cancer, Sagittarius
Onion sets	3rd or 4th	Libra, Taurus, Pisces, Cancer
Parsley	1st	Cancer, Scorpio, Pisces, Libra
Parsnips	3rd	Cancer, Scorpio, Pisces, Taurus
Peach trees	2nd or 3rd	Taurus, Libra, Virgo

Plant	Quarter	Sign
Peanuts	3rd	Cancer, Scorpio, Pisces
Pear trees	2nd or 3rd	Taurus, Libra, Virgo
Perennials	3rd	*See specific entry*
Plum trees	2nd or 3rd	Taurus, Libra, Virgo
Pole beans	1st or 2nd	Scorpio
Potatoes	3rd	Cancer, Scorpio, Taurus, Libra
Pumpkins	2nd	Cancer, Scorpio, Pisces, Libra
Quinces	1st or 2nd	Capricorn
Radishes	3rd	Libra, Taurus, Pisces, Capricorn
Rice	1st or 2nd	Scorpio
Roses	1st or 2nd	Cancer
Rutabagas	3rd	Cancer, Scorpio, Pisces, Taurus
Sage	3rd	Cancer, Scorpio, Pisces
Salsify	1st or 2nd	Cancer, Scorpio, Pisces
Spinach	1st	Cancer, Scorpio, Pisces
Squash	2nd	Cancer, Scorpio, Taurus, Libra
Strawberries	3rd	Cancer, Scorpio, Pisces
String beans	1st or 2nd	Taurus
Sunflowers	2nd, 3rd, 4th	Cancer, Libra
Tomatoes	2nd	Cancer, Scorpio, Pisces, Capricorn
Tulips	1st or 2nd	Libra, Virgo
Turnips	3rd	Cancer, Scorpio, Pisces, Taurus
Watermelon	1st or 2nd	Cancer, Scorpio, Pisces, Libra

2025 Moon Signs and Phases

Cross-reference the following month-by-month tables with the planting guide for moon phase and sign to determine the recommended planting times for 2025. Gray rows indicate the day of a phase change. All times are in Eastern Standard and Eastern Daylight Time, so be sure to adjust for your time zone.

January 2025

Date	Sign	Phase
1 Wed 5:50 am	Aquarius	1st
2 Thu	Aquarius	1st
3 Fri 10:21 am	Pisces	1st
4 Sat	Pisces	1st
5 Sun 2:01 pm	Aries	1st
6 Mon	Aries	2nd 6:56 pm
7 Tue 5:11 pm	Taurus	2nd
8 Wed	Taurus	2nd
9 Thu 8:07 pm	Gemini	2nd
10 Fri	Gemini	2nd
11 Sat 11:24 pm	Cancer	2nd
12 Sun	Cancer	2nd
13 Mon	Cancer	Full 5:27 pm
14 Tue 4:12 am	Leo	3rd
15 Wed	Leo	3rd
16 Thu 11:46 am	Virgo	3rd
17 Fri	Virgo	3rd
18 Sat 10:33 pm	Libra	3rd
19 Sun	Libra	3rd
20 Mon	Libra	3rd
21 Tue 11:20 am	Scorpio	4th 3:31 pm
22 Wed	Scorpio	4th
23 Thu 11:29 pm	Sagittarius	4th
24 Fri	Sagittarius	4th
25 Sat	Sagittarius	4th
26 Sun 8:43 am	Capricorn	4th
27 Mon	Capricorn	4th
28 Tue 2:31 pm	Aquarius	4th
29 Wed	Aquarius	New 7:36 am
30 Thu 5:52 pm	Pisces	1st
31 Fri	Pisces	1st

February 2025

Date	Sign	Phase
1 Sat 8:10 pm	Aries	1st
2 Sun	Aries	1st
3 Mon 10:33 pm	Taurus	1st
4 Tue	Taurus	1st
5 Wed	Taurus	2nd 3:02 am
6 Thu 1:44 am	Gemini	2nd
7 Fri	Gemini	2nd
8 Sat 6:04 am	Cancer	2nd
9 Sun	Cancer	2nd
10 Mon 12:01 pm	Leo	2nd
11 Tue	Leo	2nd
12 Wed 8:07 pm	Virgo	Full 8:53 am
13 Thu	Virgo	3rd
14 Fri	Virgo	3rd
15 Sat 6:45 am	Libra	3rd
16 Sun	Libra	3rd
17 Mon 7:19 pm	Scorpio	3rd
18 Tue	Scorpio	3rd
19 Wed	Scorpio	3rd
20 Thu 7:55 am	Sagittarius	4th 12:33 pm
21 Fri	Sagittarius	4th
22 Sat 6:09 pm	Capricorn	4th
23 Sun	Capricorn	4th
24 Mon	Capricorn	4th
25 Tue 12:40 am	Aquarius	4th
26 Wed	Aquarius	4th
27 Thu 3:46 am	Pisces	New 7:45 pm
28 Fri	Pisces	1st

March 2025

Date	Sign	Phase
1 Sat 4:52 am	Aries	1st
2 Sun	Aries	1st
3 Mon 5:37 am	Taurus	1st
4 Tue	Taurus	1st
5 Wed 7:29 am	Gemini	1st
6 Thu	Gemini	2nd 11:32 am
7 Fri 11:29 am	Cancer	2nd
8 Sat	Cancer	2nd
9 Sun 6:59 pm	Leo	2nd
10 Mon	Leo	2nd
11 Tue	Leo	2nd
12 Wed 3:56 am	Virgo	2nd
13 Thu	Virgo	2nd
14 Fri 2:59 pm	Libra	Full 2:55 am
15 Sat	Libra	3rd
16 Sun	Libra	3rd
17 Mon 3:30 am	Scorpio	3rd
18 Tue	Scorpio	3rd
19 Wed 4:17 pm	Sagittarius	3rd
20 Thu	Sagittarius	3rd
21 Fri	Sagittarius	3rd
22 Sat 3:29 am	Capricorn	4th 7:29 am
23 Sun	Capricorn	4th
24 Mon 11:25 am	Aquarius	4th
25 Tue	Aquarius	4th
26 Wed 3:31 pm	Pisces	4th
27 Thu	Pisces	4th
28 Fri 4:36 pm	Aries	4th
29 Sat	Aries	New 6:58 am
30 Sun 4:16 pm	Taurus	1st
31 Mon	Taurus	1st

April 2025

Date	Sign	Phase
1 Tue 4:26 pm	Gemini	1st
2 Wed	Gemini	1st
3 Thu 6:50 pm	Cancer	1st
4 Fri	Cancer	2nd 10:15 pm
5 Sat	Cancer	2nd
6 Sun 12:34 am	Leo	2nd
7 Mon	Leo	2nd
8 Tue 9:40 am	Virgo	2nd
9 Wed	Virgo	2nd
10 Thu 9:12 pm	Libra	2nd
11 Fri	Libra	2nd
12 Sat	Libra	Full 8:22 pm
13 Sun 9:54 am	Scorpio	3rd
14 Mon	Scorpio	3rd
15 Tue 10:37 pm	Sagittarius	3rd
16 Wed	Sagittarius	3rd
17 Thu	Sagittarius	3rd
18 Fri 10:12 am	Capricorn	3rd
19 Sat	Capricorn	3rd
20 Sun 7:22 pm	Aquarius	4th 9:36 pm
21 Mon	Aquarius	4th
22 Tue	Aquarius	4th
23 Wed 1:07 am	Pisces	4th
24 Thu	Pisces	4th
25 Fri 3:24 am	Aries	4th
26 Sat	Aries	4th
27 Sun 3:17 am	Taurus	New 3:31 pm
28 Mon	Taurus	1st
29 Tue 2:34 am	Gemini	1st
30 Wed	Gemini	1st

May 2025

Date	Sign	Phase
1 Thu 3:23 am	Cancer	1st
2 Fri	Cancer	1st
3 Sat 7:29 am	Leo	1st
4 Sun	Leo	2nd 9:52 am
5 Mon 3:40 pm	Virgo	2nd
6 Tue	Virgo	2nd
7 Wed	Virgo	2nd
8 Thu 3:06 am	Libra	2nd
9 Fri	Libra	2nd
10 Sat 3:58 pm	Scorpio	2nd
11 Sun	Scorpio	2nd
12 Mon	Scorpio	Full 12:56 pm
13 Tue 4:35 am	Sagittarius	3rd
14 Wed	Sagittarius	3rd
15 Thu 3:58 pm	Capricorn	3rd
16 Fri	Capricorn	3rd
17 Sat	Capricorn	3rd
18 Sun 1:29 am	Aquarius	3rd
19 Mon	Aquarius	3rd
20 Tue 8:28 am	Pisces	4th 7:59 am
21 Wed	Pisces	4th
22 Thu 12:26 pm	Aries	4th
23 Fri	Aries	4th
24 Sat 1:38 pm	Taurus	4th
25 Sun	Taurus	4th
26 Mon 1:21 pm	Gemini	New 11:02 pm
27 Tue	Gemini	1st
28 Wed 1:33 pm	Cancer	1st
29 Thu	Cancer	1st
30 Fri 4:17 pm	Leo	1st
31 Sat	Leo	1st

June 2025

Date	Sign	Phase
1 Sun 11:00 pm	Virgo	1st
2 Mon	Virgo	2nd 11:41 pm
3 Tue	Virgo	2nd
4 Wed 9:38 am	Libra	2nd
5 Thu	Libra	2nd
6 Fri 10:23 pm	Scorpio	2nd
7 Sat	Scorpio	2nd
8 Sun	Scorpio	2nd
9 Mon 10:56 am	Sagittarius	2nd
10 Tue	Sagittarius	2nd
11 Wed 9:55 pm	Capricorn	Full 3:44 am
12 Thu	Capricorn	3rd
13 Fri	Capricorn	3rd
14 Sat 7:00 am	Aquarius	3rd
15 Sun	Aquarius	3rd
16 Mon 2:09 pm	Pisces	3rd
17 Tue	Pisces	3rd
18 Wed 7:08 pm	Aries	4th 3:19 pm
19 Thu	Aries	4th
20 Fri 9:53 pm	Taurus	4th
21 Sat	Taurus	4th
22 Sun 10:57 pm	Gemini	4th
23 Mon	Gemini	4th
24 Tue 11:44 pm	Cancer	4th
25 Wed	Cancer	New 6:32 am
26 Thu	Cancer	1st
27 Fri 2:05 am	Leo	1st
28 Sat	Leo	1st
29 Sun 7:44 am	Virgo	1st
30 Mon	Virgo	1st

July 2025

Date	Sign	Phase
1 Tue 5:16 pm	Libra	1st
2 Wed	Libra	2nd 3:30 pm
3 Thu	Libra	2nd
4 Fri 5:33 am	Scorpio	2nd
5 Sat	Scorpio	2nd
6 Sun 6:06 pm	Sagittarius	2nd
7 Mon	Sagittarius	2nd
8 Tue	Sagittarius	2nd
9 Wed 4:55 am	Capricorn	2nd
10 Thu	Capricorn	Full 4:37 pm
11 Fri 1:21 pm	Aquarius	3rd
12 Sat	Aquarius	3rd
13 Sun 7:45 pm	Pisces	3rd
14 Mon	Pisces	3rd
15 Tue	Pisces	3rd
16 Wed 12:32 am	Aries	3rd
17 Thu	Aries	4th 8:38 pm
18 Fri 3:59 am	Taurus	4th
19 Sat	Taurus	4th
20 Sun 6:22 am	Gemini	4th
21 Mon	Gemini	4th
22 Tue 8:26 am	Cancer	4th
23 Wed	Cancer	4th
24 Thu 11:28 am	Leo	New 3:11 pm
25 Fri	Leo	1st
26 Sat 4:55 pm	Virgo	1st
27 Sun	Virgo	1st
28 Mon	Virgo	1st
29 Tue 1:43 am	Libra	1st
30 Wed	Libra	1st
31 Thu 1:25 pm	Scorpio	1st

August 2025

Date	Sign	Phase
1 Fri	Scorpio	2nd 8:41 am
2 Sat	Scorpio	2nd
3 Sun 2:00 am	Sagittarius	2nd
4 Mon	Sagittarius	2nd
5 Tue 1:04 pm	Capricorn	2nd
6 Wed	Capricorn	2nd
7 Thu 9:18 pm	Aquarius	2nd
8 Fri	Aquarius	2nd
9 Sat	Aquarius	Full 3:55 am
10 Sun 2:50 am	Pisces	3rd
11 Mon	Pisces	3rd
12 Tue 6:33 am	Aries	3rd
13 Wed	Aries	3rd
14 Thu 9:22 am	Taurus	3rd
15 Fri	Taurus	3rd
16 Sat 12:01 pm	Gemini	4th 1:12 am
17 Sun	Gemini	4th
18 Mon 3:05 pm	Cancer	4th
19 Tue	Cancer	4th
20 Wed 7:17 pm	Leo	4th
21 Thu	Leo	4th
22 Fri	Leo	4th
23 Sat 1:24 am	Virgo	New 2:07 am
24 Sun	Virgo	1st
25 Mon 10:08 am	Libra	1st
26 Tue	Libra	1st
27 Wed 9:27 pm	Scorpio	1st
28 Thu	Scorpio	1st
29 Fri	Scorpio	1st
30 Sat 10:04 am	Sagittarius	1st
31 Sun	Sagittarius	2nd 2:25 am

September 2025

Date	Sign	Phase
1 Mon 9:45 pm	Capricorn	2nd
2 Tue	Capricorn	2nd
3 Wed	Capricorn	2nd
4 Thu 6:32 am	Aquarius	2nd
5 Fri	Aquarius	2nd
6 Sat 11:54 am	Pisces	2nd
7 Sun	Pisces	Full 2:09 pm
8 Mon 2:37 pm	Aries	3rd
9 Tue	Aries	3rd
10 Wed 4:03 pm	Taurus	3rd
11 Thu	Taurus	3rd
12 Fri 5:38 pm	Gemini	3rd
13 Sat	Gemini	3rd
14 Sun 8:30 pm	Cancer	4th 6:33 am
15 Mon	Cancer	4th
16 Tue	Cancer	4th
17 Wed 1:20 am	Leo	4th
18 Thu	Leo	4th
19 Fri 8:23 am	Virgo	4th
20 Sat	Virgo	4th
21 Sun 5:41 pm	Libra	New 3:54 pm
22 Mon	Libra	1st
23 Tue	Libra	1st
24 Wed 5:00 am	Scorpio	1st
25 Thu	Scorpio	1st
26 Fri 5:37 pm	Sagittarius	1st
27 Sat	Sagittarius	1st
28 Sun	Sagittarius	1st
29 Mon 5:55 am	Capricorn	2nd 7:54 pm
30 Tue	Capricorn	2nd

October 2025

Date	Sign	Phase
1 Wed 3:52 pm	Aquarius	2nd
2 Thu	Aquarius	2nd
3 Fri 10:07 pm	Pisces	2nd
4 Sat	Pisces	2nd
5 Sun	Pisces	2nd
6 Mon 12:48 am	Aries	Full 11:48 pm
7 Tue	Aries	3rd
8 Wed 1:12 am	Taurus	3rd
9 Thu	Taurus	3rd
10 Fri 1:12 am	Gemini	3rd
11 Sat	Gemini	3rd
12 Sun 2:37 am	Cancer	3rd
13 Mon	Cancer	4th 2:13 pm
14 Tue 6:47 am	Leo	4th
15 Wed	Leo	4th
16 Thu 2:06 pm	Virgo	4th
17 Fri	Virgo	4th
18 Sat	Virgo	4th
19 Sun 12:01 am	Libra	4th
20 Mon	Libra	4th
21 Tue 11:42 am	Scorpio	New 8:25 am
22 Wed	Scorpio	1st
23 Thu	Scorpio	1st
24 Fri 12:19 am	Sagittarius	1st
25 Sat	Sagittarius	1st
26 Sun 12:53 pm	Capricorn	1st
27 Mon	Capricorn	1st
28 Tue 11:55 pm	Aquarius	1st
29 Wed	Aquarius	2nd 12:21 pm
30 Thu	Aquarius	2nd
31 Fri 7:46 am	Pisces	2nd

November 2025

Date	Sign	Phase
1 Sat	Pisces	2nd
2 Sun 10:39 am	Aries	2nd
3 Mon	Aries	2nd
4 Tue 11:16 am	Taurus	2nd
5 Wed	Taurus	Full 8:19 am
6 Thu 10:20 am	Gemini	3rd
7 Fri	Gemini	3rd
8 Sat 10:06 am	Cancer	3rd
9 Sun	Cancer	3rd
10 Mon 12:34 pm	Leo	3rd
11 Tue	Leo	3rd
12 Wed 6:52 pm	Virgo	4th 12:28 am
13 Thu	Virgo	4th
14 Fri	Virgo	4th
15 Sat 4:44 am	Libra	4th
16 Sun	Libra	4th
17 Mon 4:44 pm	Scorpio	4th
18 Tue	Scorpio	4th
19 Wed	Scorpio	4th
20 Thu 5:26 am	Sagittarius	New 1:47 am
21 Fri	Sagittarius	1st
22 Sat 5:53 pm	Capricorn	1st
23 Sun	Capricorn	1st
24 Mon	Capricorn	1st
25 Tue 5:16 am	Aquarius	1st
26 Wed	Aquarius	1st
27 Thu 2:24 pm	Pisces	1st
28 Fri	Pisces	2nd 1:59 am
29 Sat 8:07 pm	Aries	2nd
30 Sun	Aries	2nd

December 2025

Date	Sign	Phase
1 Mon 10:13 pm	Taurus	2nd
2 Tue	Taurus	2nd
3 Wed 9:48 pm	Gemini	2nd
4 Thu	Gemini	Full 6:14 pm
5 Fri 8:54 pm	Cancer	3rd
6 Sat	Cancer	3rd
7 Sun 9:48 pm	Leo	3rd
8 Mon	Leo	3rd
9 Tue	Leo	3rd
10 Wed 2:20 am	Virgo	3rd
11 Thu	Virgo	4th 3:52 pm
12 Fri 11:04 am	Libra	4th
13 Sat	Libra	4th
14 Sun 10:51 pm	Scorpio	4th
15 Mon	Scorpio	4th
16 Tue	Scorpio	4th
17 Wed 11:38 am	Sagittarius	4th
18 Thu	Sagittarius	4th
19 Fri 11:53 pm	Capricorn	New 8:43 pm
20 Sat	Capricorn	1st
21 Sun	Capricorn	1st
22 Mon 10:52 am	Aquarius	1st
23 Tue	Aquarius	1st
24 Wed 8:09 pm	Pisces	1st
25 Thu	Pisces	1st
26 Fri	Pisces	1st
27 Sat 3:02 am	Aries	2nd 2:10 pm
28 Sun	Aries	2nd
29 Mon 6:57 am	Taurus	2nd
30 Tue	Taurus	2nd
31 Wed 8:13 am	Gemini	2nd

Contributors

Anne Sala is a freelance journalist in Minnesota. As her two children grow, she is happily making room for them to work alongside her in the kitchen. Their help is particularly welcomed when making the sweetly spiced pies that accompany holiday meals.

Bonnie Rose Weaver is a clinical herbalist, educator, and artist based on the traditional lands of the Ramaytush Ohlone people, modern-day San Francisco, CA. They are passionate about connecting plants and people through increasing access to and education about herbs. Learn more about their work and current offerings at bonnieroseweaver.com and @bonnieroseweaver.

Charlie Rainbow Wolf is happiest when she is creating something, especially if it's made from items that others have discarded. A recorded singer-songwriter and published author, she champions holistic living and lives in the Midwest with her husband and special-needs Great Danes. Astrology reports, smoke cleansing blends, and more are available through her website at charlierainbow.com.

Diana Rajchel is an animistic witch who interacts with spirits cultivated and uncultivated. As a result, people ask her for spirit work when they discover roommates they weren't aware they had consented to. She is the co-owner of Golden Apple Metaphysical with Nikki Jobin and the author of *Urban Magick* and *Hex Twisting*. Book her for consultations or see what she's come up with this time at dianarajchel.com.

Elizabeth Barrette lives in central Illinois and enjoys magical crafts, historic religions, and gardening for wildlife. She has written columns on Pagan practice, speculative fiction, gender studies, and social and environmental issues. Her book *Composing Magic* explains how to combine writing and spirituality. Visit her blog at ysabetwordsmith.dreamwidth.org.

Geoffrey Edwards is a healing arts practitioner whose practice encompasses art therapy, herbalism, and community acupuncture. He is the owner of Grain & Pestle, an apothecary, clinic, and art therapy studio based in Detroit, MI. Geoffrey has facilitated plant walks and workshops on numerous topics, including ecology, the elements, mental health, and the expressive therapies.

Herbalist, author, and international speaker **Holly Bellebuono** has been teaching herbal medicine for thirty years. She directs the Bellebuono School of Herbal Medicine with online and in-person programs, retreats, and herbal certifications. She is also a business coach and directs the Selle Entrepreneur Network, an online community for creative women. Visit HollyBellebuono .com to learn more and enroll.

Iya Angelique "Sobande" Greer has degrees in communications, public relations, and health and nutrition and is also a certified natural health professional and a holistic health consultant. Iya Sobande's products, services, workshops, and literary publications have been featured in a variety of magazines, radio shows, and other publications over the past thirty years. She currently teaches and assists clients at her private practice near Nashville, TN.

James Kambos is a writer, artist, and herbalist. He's written many articles on folk magic and herbs. He raises herbs and wildflowers in his southern Ohio garden.

JD Walker is an avid student of herbalism and gardening. She has written a regular garden column for thirty years. She is an award-winning author, journalist, and magazine editor and a frequent contributor to the Llewellyn annuals. Her first book, *A Witch's Guide to Wildcrafting*, published by Llewellyn Publications, was released in spring 2021. Her new book, *Under the Sacred Canopy*, is out now.

Jill Henderson is a backwoods herbalist, author, artist, and world traveler with a penchant for wild edible and medicinal plants, culinary herbs, and nature ecology. She is a longtime contributor to *Llewellyn's Herbal Almanac* and *Acres USA* magazine and is the author of *The Healing Power of Kitchen Herbs, A Journey of Seasons*, and *The Garden Seed Saving Guide*. Visit Jill's blog at ShowMeOz.wordpress.com.

Jordan Charbonneau is a homesteader, hiker, animal lover, and forager. She attended Sterling College (Vermont), where she double-majored in ecology and environmental humanities. Today, Jordan lives in a little off-grid cabin she and her husband, Scott, built in the hills of West Virginia. Together they grow organic vegetables and care for tons of animals. You can keep up with her writing on the Southern Exposure Seed Exchange blog and her own blog, rabbitridgefarmwv.com.

Kathy Martin is the longtime author of the blog *Skippy's Vegetable Garden*, a journal of her vegetable gardens, which has won awards including *Horticulture Magazine*'s Best Gardening Blog. She helps run Aurelia's Garden Inc., a nonprofit microfarm that donates to food pantries. Kathy is a Master Gardener and a retired biomedical researcher who lives near Boston with her family, dogs, chickens, and honeybees.

Linda Raedisch has written four books of nonfiction, including *The Secret History of Christmas Baking: Recipes and Stories from Tomb Offerings to Gingerbread Boys* (Llewellyn, 2023). You can follow her dubious kitchen, gardening, and writing adventures on Instagram @lindaraedisch.

Lupa is an author, artist, and naturalist Pagan in the Pacific Northwest. She has written several books on nature-based Paganism and is the creator of the *Tarot of Bones*. A lifelong creative, her more recent efforts involve rediscovering her love of traditional illustration. Find out more about Lupa and her work at thegreenwolf.com.

Mandana Boushee is an Iranian-American community herbalist, a storyteller, a land tender, and a joyous member of the mycelial network of liberatory creators and lovers. She is a cofounder and educator at Wild Gather, School of Herbal Studies. Through her shared wisdom and initiatives in the Mahicantuck (Hudson) Valley, she works to offer her community access to equitable care, plant medicine, and herbal education.

Mason Olonade is a father, farmer, artist, and husband in Charlotte, NC. Professionally trained as a molecular biologist, his study of life continues through his work as a volunteer farmer in Charlotte, and with the Family Pattern Project at the Pattern House of Olonade. Whether working with disadvantaged youth in the cornfields or with clients at his studio, he cultivates the most important crop, the *n'krabea*, or destiny, with care.

Marilyn I. Bellemore, a teacher and author, recently moved back to a farm in the Green Mountains of central Vermont. She continues to preserve fruits and flowers in a variety of jellies, jams, syrups, and butters. Marilyn's love of herbs is predominate in her gardens, her studies, and the bath and body products that she enjoys making. She is currently renovating her farmhouse in East Point, Prince Edward Island, Canada.

Mireille Blacke, RD, CD-N, is a licensed alcohol and drug counselor, registered dietitian, and freelance health and nutrition writer from the Hartford, Connecticut, area. She has written numerous articles for Llewellyn's annuals since 2014. Mireille worked in rock radio for two decades before shifting her career focus to media psychology, behavioral health nutrition, and addiction counseling. Her Bengal cats consume most of her free time and sanity.

Monica Crosson is the author of *A Year in the Enchanted Garden*, *Wild Magical Soul*, *The Magickal Family*, and *Summer Sage*. She is a Master Gardener who lives in the beautiful Pacific Northwest, happily digging in the dirt and tending her raspberries with her family and their small menagerie of farm animals. Monica is a regular contributor to Llewellyn's annuals as well as *Enchanted Living Magazine* and *Witchology Magazine*.

Natalie Zaman is the author of *Color and Conjure* and *Magical Destinations of the Northeast*. A regular contributor to various Llewellyn annual publications, she also writes the recurring feature Wandering Witch for *Witches & Pagans* magazine. When not on the road, she's busy tending her magical back garden. Visit Natalie online at nataliezaman.blogspot.com.

Rachael Witt is a clinical community herbalist, gardener, and teacher. She is the founder of Wildness Within, an herbal business that offers plant-focused apprenticeships and classes, herbal consultations, and handmade remedies. Rachael is dedicated to simple, seasonal living with the land and teaching people hands-on-earth skills. She lives and stewards the Highlands Homestead in Duvall, Washington. Find more at Wildness-WithinLiving.com.

Rebecca Gilbert discovered her love of foraging at age six when she spent the summer with her grandmother in Martha's Vineyard, Massachusetts. She has been exploring the subject—and grazing on the same farm—ever since. She teaches a variety of rural skills at Native Earth Teaching Farm, which she and her husband opened to the public in 2002.

Sara Mellas is an artist and writer living in Nashville, TN. She's authored three books and written about food, music, comedy, and astrology for several media outlets. She holds a master's degree in music education and vocal performance and works as a performer and food stylist for television, commercials, and live events. Her website is saramellas.com.

Susan Pesznecker is a mother, writer, nurse, and college English professor living in the beautiful Pacific Northwest with her poodles. An amateur herbalist, Sue loves reading, writing, cooking, travel, and anything having to do with the outdoors. Her previous works include *Crafting Magick with Pen and Ink, The Magickal Retreat*, and *Yule*. She's a regular contributor to the Llewellyn annuals. Follow her on Instagram at @SusanPesznecker.

Gardening Resources

Cooking with Herbs and Spices compiled by **Susan Pesznecker**
Gardening Techniques written by **Jill Henderson**
2025 Themed Garden Plans designed by **Laurel Woodward**
2025 Gardening Log tips written by **Natalie Zaman**